GRIGORI GRABOVOI

PATENTS FOR INVENTIONS

Hamburg 2011

Jelezky publishing

www.jelezky-media.com

1. Edition

English first edition, april 2011

© 2011 english first edition

Dimitri Eletski, Hamburg (Editor)

Further information about the contents:

SVET centre, Hamburg

www.svet-centre.eu

GRIGORI GRABOVOI

PATENTS FOR INVENTIONS

ISBN: 978-3-00-034093-2

CONTENTS

Scientific and Technical Collection "ELECTRONIC TECHNOLOGY", series 3 "MICROELECTRONICS", Volume 1 (153), 1999, Central Scientific Research Institute "Elektronika", Moscow.
Article by Grigori Grabovoi (aka Grabovoi Grigori Petrovich, aka G.P. Grabovoi) "Исследование и анализ фундаментальных определений" ["Studies and Analysis of the Basic Definitions"].

ELECTRONIC

TECHNOLOGY

series 3

MICROELECTRONICS

volume 1(153)

1999

Scientific and Technical Collection "ELECTRONIC TECHNOLOGY", series 3 "MICROELECTRONICS", Volume 1 (153), 1999, Central Scientific Research Institute "Elektronika", Moscow.
Article by Grigori Grabovoi "Studies and Analysis of the Basic Definitions".

Ministry of Economics of the Russian Federation
Department of Radio Electronics and Instrument
Engineering

ELECTRONIC TECHNOLOGY

Series 3

MICROELECTRONICS

Volume 1 (153)
Scientific and Technical Collection   1999   Published since 1965

CONTENTS

Central Scientific Research Institute "Elektronika"
Moscow

Electronic Technology. Series 3. Microelectronics. Vol. 1 (153), 1999

BIOFIELD ELECTRONICS

From the Editorial Board

We are opening the new column with an article by Grigori Grabovoi, the founder of a new science and technology direction – biofield electronics, and specifically forecast-oriented control of microprocesses. Nature has generously endowed Grigori Grabovoi with unique abilities of a clairvoyant, which he has enriched by relying on knowledge he received at the Applied Mathematics and Mechanics Department of Tashkent State University and applied to control of events. The practical experience of control of events he has accumulated Grigori Grabovoi uses in the interest of people's safety – my and your safety and safety of the country; he has worked as an adviser to the Federal Aviation Authority of Russia and a consultant of the Security Council of the Russian Federation and Ministry of Civil Defense, Emergencies and Disaster Relief of the Russian Federation, diagnosing nuclear power plants, submarines, military facilities and government aircraft to identify possible troubles and accidents.

The Grigori Grabovoi article describes physical and mathematical models of the mechanism of forming forecast-oriented information (clairvoyance) and control of events based on information derived about future events. In doing this he relies on the well-known principle of dialectical materialism stating that we live in a cause-and-effect world. This makes it possible to draw the following conclusions:

- for each cause that has occurred in the past there is a corresponding effect realized in the future;
- to change the effect it is necessary to change the cause;
- to control events it is necessary and sufficient to affect the cause – to change or eliminate it.

Having learned to control events and having started applying his knowledge to practice, Grigori Grabovoi understood the need of people and society as a whole for such activity the goal of which is to save people's lives and prevent anthropogenic catastrophes. One person alone cannot handle the scope of work, and Grigori Grabovoi, following the logic of a creative scientist, decided to use technical means for this purpose and developed a crystal module. The instrument principle of operation is based on the property of some crystals to split a laser beam into two beams, one beam carrying information about the future (effects) and the other beam carrying information about the past (causes). And one can change information about the past changing the arrangement of crystals using the method of calculation developed by Grigori Grabovoi. Lastly, he has developed a tutorial for training specialists in forecast and control of events, particularly in diagnostics and control of the industrial process of manufacturing of integrated circuits (IC). When manufacturing of the next batch of IC is launched, these specialists will be able to receive cause-and-effect information about its course and take measures ahead of time to eliminate the causes that can result in rejects, and thus to achieve the percentage yield as specified in technical documentation, i.e., to develop a forecast-oriented quality system of IC development and manufacturing. Earlier, Grigori Grabovoi taught diagnostics and control of events to test pilots, cosmonauts, and operators of nuclear power plants and other facilities. This characterizes Grigori Grabovoi as a distinguished scientist who has created not just a new field of science, but also his own school of science.

To facilitate understanding of the presented material it is recommended that the reader start reading the article beginning from the part devoted to the description of the crystal module.

Deputy Editor-in-Chief Professor Garyainov S.A., DTS [Doctor of Technical Sciences]

Scientific and Technical Collection "ELECTRONIC TECHNOLOGY", series 3 "MICROELECTRONICS", Volume 1 (153), 1999, Central Scientific Research Institute "Elektronika", Moscow.
Article by Grigori Grabovoi "Studies and Analysis of the Basic Definitions".

Elerctronic Technology. Series 3. Microelectronics. Vol. 1 (153), 1999

GRIGORI GRABOVOI

Grigori Grabovoi

Graduated from Tashkent State University, Applied Mathematics and Physics Department, a Corresponding Member of the RAEN [Russian Academy of Natural Sciences], an Active member of the MAI [International Informatization Academy]. The author of original works on forecast, control and correction of future events and on fundamentals of calculation and development of equipment (instruments) designed for the above purposes. Based on these works, Grigori Grabovoi identifies impending catastrophes thus saving people from death, forecasts earthquakes and, using a crystal module, the instrument he developed, warns 14 days in advance of possible destruction in the earthquake zone where the instruments are installed. As an adviser to the Federal Aviation Authority of Russia and a consultant of the Security Council of the Russian Federation and Ministry of Civil Defense, Emergencies and Disaster Relief of the Russian Federation, Grigori Grabovoi diagnoses nuclear power plants and government aircraft to identify possible troubles and accidents.

For graduate students of the Department of Cause-and-Effect Quality System (CEQS) Grigori Grabovoi will teach a course on forecast and control of events and conduct training and certification of graduate students on the ability to use cause-and-effect information for control of industrial processes and for business management.

"Science Center" Graduate School

Scientific and Technical Collection "ELECTRONIC TECHNOLOGY", series 3 "MICROELECTRONICS", Volume 1 (153), 1999, Central Scientific Research Institute "Elektronika", Moscow.
Article by Grigori Grabovoi "Studies and Analysis of the Basic Definitions".

GRIGORI GRABOVOI

STUDIES AND ANALYSIS OF FUNDAMENTAL DEFINITIONS OF OPTICAL SYSTEMS IN PREVENTION OF CATASTROPHES AND FORECAST-ORIENTED CONTROL OF MICRO-PROCESSES

The work was performed using the auhtor's method for digital analysis of form of information.

Relevance

The relevance of the work is that a physical and mathematical theory and an intrument for forecasting catastrophic phenomena have been developed which make it possible to identify the component of information pertaining to future events. Because a lot of natural and anthropogenic catastrophic events occur with no statistical and deterministic basis, the work is especially relevant in discoveries aimed at acquiring accurate information about future time, including methods for prevention of catastrophes.

In the work, principles of theoretical and instrument technologies that are built based on the postulate of interconnections of all elements of reality are realized [1]. Also, a structural analytical approach to building control systems wherein each component performs the task of harmonic development of all components of reality is defined. A method for producing a substance based on extracting matter by using a mechanism for control of the zone of future events is demonstrated. Using this technology it is possible to place individual control pulses of current time into crystals so as to obtain the required substance at the predetermined point of future space and time.

Subject of the studies:
earthquakes, industrial facilities, any reality with known or unknown parameters.

The scientific novelty of the studies is that:
-        for the first time a method for extracting information about future events has been realized the-oretically and practically;
-        for the first time an approach has been used when control of any object of information takes place in the current coordinate of acquiring information about the object's properties;
-        a principle of precise control of objects of reality with characteristics that are either unknown or cannot be determined in a timely manner has been realized.

The theoretical importance of the studies lies in:
-        the fundamental definitions of optical systems;

- generalizations and effects of the definitions; and
- the development of structural-analytical technologies of prevention and forecast of catastrophes, and first of all of catastrophes that threaten the entire world.

The practical importance of the studies lies in:
- the instrument for prevention and forecast of catastrophes of industrial facilities that was developed using methods of computer simulation, and the development of a new direction of control of microprocessors;
- expansion of the results to any object of reality;
- deriving methodological principles of building anthropogenic systems harmonized with respect to any environment.

Testing and Implementation of the Results

The testing and implementation of the results were conducted using the author's technology of digital analysis of form of information extracted for any object based on the principle of interconnections of all information units [2]. Based on personal experience of precise control using

irrational methods and principles of transferring the results of such control to material structures described in the doctoral thesis "Applied Structures of the Creating Information Field", numerical data were developed that determine the correctness of the structural-analytical mechanism of operation and include theoretical and practical results. As the source material for digital analysis of the instrument operation from the standpoint of correspondence to real processes, data on monitoring Earth's surface from planet satellites by means of control systems provided by the Agency for Monitoring and Forecasting Emergency Situations (VNII GOChS [All-Russia Scientific Research Institute on Problems of Civil Defense and Emergency Situations]) of the Ministry of Civil Defense, Emergencies and Disaster Relief of Russia were used.

1.

1. Introduction

Studies of processes of reality taking into account the fact that future events are recognizable in current events make it possible to prevent catastrophes and control future events. The essence of this approach is that events of the future are viewed from the present in the form of controlled structures [3]. The information of future events is identified through areas of transition from the future to the present. The transition areas are constructed on seven coordinates: three coordinates of the current time space, the time coordinate, two coordinates of time intervals for the past and the future, and the object response coordinate. In the general case, the object response coordinate denotes the area of interaction of

8

all objects of information, and in a particular case it can mean a person's perception. To save an object of information from destruction, one can use transformation of the interval of future time through past time, projecting the data into the three-dimensional space of current time. Optical systems meet the requirements of signal recording. When moving through the optical medium of crystals, an element of light splits into components corresponding to all areas of information.

A light component organized in the form of reflection of future events through the interval of the past is a point that, as far as its properties are concerned, is infinitely distant from but physically is inside the crystal, which makes it possible to describe properties of the optical system based on recording and decoding of events of the future. Having thus a fragment of future processes in current time it is possible to construct matter of the future in accordance with the harmonic phase of development and with required precision. Knowing the distribution of signals from the future in the area of control of reality it is possible to prevent catastrophes by developing an optical system that harmonizes all areas of information. It is light signals that are processed because light has the property of splitting in crystals into the components of current and future time. One can see the physical meaning of this phenomenon in a model form if one considers properties in the time interval < 10-17 s. Then, the information segment corresponding to future time for the time interval > 10-12 s can be viewed as an element adjacent to the information segment corresponding to current time. The interface of the segments of future and current time can be expressed physically by means of a crystal system. Because of this, the system splits light into the elements of current and future time. This means that by specifying parameters of the optical system that is built based on the laws of crystalline structure it is possible to control mater and create elements of events in the required manner.

2.   *The Fundamental Definitions of Optical Systems*

The fundamental definitions of optical systems are defined in three areas.

2.1   The first area is the definition of informational interaction of objects in future time for the initial space and for perception of current time.

2.1.1   The formulation and information of discovering energy of the future.

Energy of the future has been defined: it consists of energy of the past multiplied by the space of distribution of energy of current time and divided by space of distribution of energy of the past:

$$\Psi = \frac{E \cdot W}{U}, \qquad\qquad (1)$$

where Ψ is energy of the future, E is energy of the past, W is the space of distribution of energy of current time, and U is the space of distribution of energy of past time.

The novelty of the definition of energy of the future is that for the first time a segment of energy of future objects of information that makes it possible to determine the future from the desired values has been isolated.

The field of application of the definition is realizable in all control systems and systems for optical conversion of information. In optical systems built on crystals, light splitting is registered in accordance with the discovery of energy of the future.

Ψ is derived by determining the space of crystals in W, the space of the area of measurement in U, and E as energy of the emitted light pulse. The control forecast is set based on the classification of Ψ depending on the norm of events.

2.2   The second area is the definition of energy of the past.

2.2.1   The formulation and data for the definition of energy of the past.

Energy of the past is determined in the form of the product of energy of current time (energy of the present) and the functions of intersection of energies of the future and the past:

$$E = E_{\text{н}} \cdot F, \qquad (2)$$

where E is energy of the present, and F is the function of intersection of energies of the future and the past.

The novelty of the definition of energy of the past is that previously unknown phenomena of reality have been discovered that make it possible to determine in one area energies of all times.

The field of application of energy of the past is realized in systems of recognition of signals from objects located in any reality, including reality with an unknown structure. Conceptually, F is identified with Ψ. Signal recognition in the structure of crystal optical systems is realized by fixing F in areas of interaction of signals between crystals.

2.3   The third area is the definition of common reality.

2.3.1   The formulation and data for the definition of common reality.

Reality that is common to all processes has been defined; its essence is that a pulse of any event converts to current time (to events of the present) in the area of intersection of the past and the future. As a result, the reality of any process is converted in the area of remote and unique content to a reproducible environment, i.e., any process is as unique as the frequency of its repetition in the area of energy conversion to the present (to events of current time). Therefore, any element of reality in the conversion phase is indestructible and repeatable under any conditions of the internal and external environment. So, any element of reality can be restored. In a formalized form the discovery formulae are presented as follows:

$$W = \frac{\Psi \cdot W1(W)}{E_{\text{ч}}}, \qquad (3)$$

where W is common reality, and W1 is the function of common reality for recorded phenomena of any environment.

The novelty of the definition of common reality is that for the first time the functional environment has been defined that makes it possible to convert and describe any processes of reality from one point.

The field of application of the definition of common reality in optoconducting systems makes it possible to isolate the converting pulse of any environment and to control reality. In the general case, the discovery determines all phenomena of reality.

3.   The Effects and Generalizations of the Definitions

The effect of the fundamental definitions of optical systems is practical realization of laws of control optical pulse.

The first law is that crystal-based optical systems are reproducible as a reflection of future events through a picoseconds interval of the past.

The second law is the movement of an optical signal both in the direction of recording systems and into an environment of indefinable properties. As a result, it is possible to identify the information constant that determines control of environments with unknown structure.

The third law is that the use of the area of projection of the future onto the present as the basis of pulse difference for various environments determines the structure of the instrument that harmonizes all systems.

The fourth law is that a system definable by an optical signal is always definable for processes of an infinite series. The corollary of the fourth law is that all processes of reality are described in each of its areas. This is why the world responds to changes when there are already no more changes in the world. There is only eternity that consists of itself. The next corollary is that eternity of a crystal is a reflection of the reality that is taking place.

The generalization of the fundamental definitions of optical systems determines the mechanism of connection of the formal apparatus of discoveries with the phenomena of the internal and external environment. Generalization of the discovery of energy of the future makes it possible to determine the future in the reflection of a segment of future events on the environment that has considerable temperature differentials or to determine the form of a crystal system.

Detalization of objects of reality combined with simultaneous generalization of the control environment leads to wave synthesis systems. The essence of a wave synthesis system in describing processes of reality is that reality is viewed as periodic intersection of stationary and dynamic areas. In the area of intersections, synthesis of the dynamic and stationary waves of reality occurs. By identifying the dynamic phase in a stationary area, infinite functioning of the stationary area is achieved. In crystals, a similar process makes it possible, by solving the inverse problem, to derive from the stationary environment (from the crystal)

11

the dynamic component of wave synthesis, i.e., the time phase. In description of reality the theory of wave synthesis is formally expressed as follows:

$$T = Y \cdot S, \qquad\qquad (4)$$

where T is time, Y is the wave of the dynamic phase of reality, and S is the stationary phase of reality.

In a certain case, wave synthesis of reality can be imagined as an infinite wave that periodically passes stationary areas and creates new phases of reality from intersection processes. Fixing the dynamic phase component in the stationary phase makes it possible to make the stationary phase time-independent - virtually eternal. Consequently, for such area the created object is eternal and hence always recoverable [4]. Considering earthquakes from this position it is possible, through reflections on faces of crystals, to derive the criterion of recoverability of the measurement environment in time. This criterion makes it possible to accurately determine the time of earthquake origination. For a human being, the theory of wave synthesis proves immortality. According to the theory of wave synthesis, in order to realize immortality it is necessary to convert the area of reproduction of the stationary phase of reality S to the wave of the dynamic phase of reality Y.

One of the indicators of such conversion is reproduction of genes from human thoughts-forms. This is why in systems of optical recognition and control of an earthquake the potentially eternal system, "a human", interacts with a system of crystals in the area of reproduction of the stationary phase. Such interaction not only forecasts an earthquake, but also harmonically reduces its magnitude. Recorded is the earthquake with the already reduced magnitude. So an instrument for forecasting an earthquake that is built on an optical medium has the function of harmonic reduction or complete prevention of an earthquake. Herein, information about an earthquake that did not happen is not reproduced anywhere else, and it even prolongs the life of the instrument. In this case, potential eternity of a human being practically reproduces the life of the instrument. The eternal begets eternal. In generalized sense, all instruments and mechanisms that are reproduced by humans must satisfy the described conditions. Then, according to the feedback principle, these instruments and mechanisms will always be creative for humans, and under no conditions will they destroy not just humans, but also the environment. To build such technology it is necessary to transfer the laws of propagation of optical signals to the design and operating principles of technical systems.

Studies of optical media in the direction of separation of phases of optical pulse are conducted using the principle of minimizing resistance of the medium along the pulse trajectory. In a particular case this means separation of the motion vector along which the absorption factor is minimal. In a system of common connections where each object interacts with all other objects, including the objects of the future and the past, the optical element of current time splits a light pulse into three time phases. According to the theory of wave synthesis, one can view current time as a dynamic wave, time of the past as a static area, and time of the future as a synthesized phase of reality built by fixing the static area in the dynamic wave. Creation of a known substance takes place through the static area, and creation of an unknown substance takes place during the initial period of synthesis of future reality. For optical systems, the event-driven part that corresponds to time for the past is defined as an optical medium with fixed characteristics (for instance, a crystal), for current time – by a light pulse, and for the future – by the synthesized area that arises from light pulse interaction with the crystal. According to the stated distribution, the formula of energy of the future $\Psi = E \cdot W/U$ means that events of the future based on energy of the future Ψ are determined by the fixed value of elapsed light pulse E under the conditions when U denotes the optical system space, and W denotes the space of the optical system and measurement areas. Taking into account the fact that from the formula of energy of the past $E = E_{\text{н}} \cdot F$, energy of the present $E_{\text{н}}$ is determined by the current (changeable) value of a light pulse, one can derive function F in the form of projection of measurement areas on the analytical system of optical media. The analytical system of optical media is located in space P that comprises an optical medium with fixed properties, and an optical medium comprising changing areas of intersection and reflection of light pulses. Using the fact that from the formula of common reality

$$\Psi \cdot W1(W)/E_{\text{н}}$$

one can determine characteristics of events from one point, we derive W1(W) for space P in the form of projection of measurement areas on P. Taking into account W, in the method for measurement the optical medium first creatively and harmonically redefines reality to reduce the earthquake magnitude or to prevent the earthquake, and then determines the earthquake parameters. In the general case, using the expression for W it is possible to convert information about any catastrophes toward reduction or prevention. According to the law of common connections between all phenomena of reality, the results derived for optical systems can be transferred to any media that have similar functions. It follows that measurements and prevention of catastrophic phenomena of reality can be performed from any point of reality. If the control forecast of phenomena of reality which means reduction or prevention of catastrophes is built by means of an optical system-based instrument, then the instrument functions are determined by the criteria of light pulses.

5. Structural-Analytical Instruments for Prevention of Earthquakes and Catastrophes

Using the structure of optical systems derived in this work which makes it possible to harmonically forecast and prevent catastrophes, one can build instruments that, when used, do not cause any negative consequences in any time or space [5]. A catastrophe that is prevented or has reduced magnitude by means of such instruments is already not realized anywhere. Equipment and any facilities that are created must be built using this harmonization principle. Such technology is safe for the producer and the environment.

A Crystal Module for Forecasting Earthquakes and Catastrophes. Module Functions in Creating Substance

Earthquakes can be forecast in the interval from one to seven days by using aligned crystals. The arrangement of crystals made of rock crystal (chemical composition - quartz, trigonal crystal scheme, hardness 7,0, specific weight 2,65, refraction 1,54-1,55, birefringence 0,009) in the projection along coordinate planes is as follows:
over area ZOX (OX is the horizontal axis, and OZ is the vertical axis)

1 2 3 4 5 6 7 8 9 10 11 12 13 14 15 16 17 18 19 20 21 22

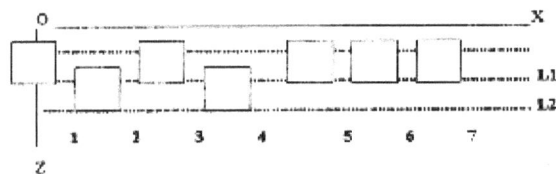

The arrangement of crystals is shown on the diagram. Each crystal is a cube with a 3 cm long side. The cubes are located on plane ZOX. One side of the cubes 1, 3, 5, 6, 7 is on straight line L1, and of cubes 2 and 4 – on straight line L2. The distance between straight lines L1 and L2 is 1,5 cm, and they are parallel to axis OX. The distance between crystals 4 and 5 is 2 cm, and the distance between the other crystals is 1 cm. The crystals are located in a transparent sphere. Characteristics of the crystals and the sphere must satisfy the conditions of splitting a light pulse from a map of the terrain along two projections. The condition of splitting a light pulse includes the principle of amplification of its projections due to signals reflected from the surfaces. The device principle is based on the fact that when converting light in special optical medium, the separation of the light pulse form that corresponds to future events occurs. The crystal arrangement is chosen such that prevention of earthquakes and catastrophes occurs, with harmonization of creative development of the future in plus/minus infinity. This device is built with realization of the concept of creative properties of any technical device. Output characteristics of light make it possible to acquire information about an earthquake time and magnitude for the period of seven future days. For an instrument with rock crystal as the material of crystal cubes, the cube surfaces must be as flat as possible, with the micrometer finish accuracy. Absorption of a monochromatic wave with a $4,3 \cdot 10^{-7}$ wavelength by the surface during a nanosecond pulse must

14

be equal to 0,5 with reflectance of the map of the terrain equal to 0,62. It is necessary to change surface properties during periods of time that correspond to the instrument life. The instrument life can be increased multifold by adding an external optical lens to it. It will be necessary to calculate the change of the lens position every five months after the first nine months of instrument operation. After the first three five-month periods, four-month periods are calculated three times and so on, until ten-day periods. Then, it is necessary to change the lens shape. Output parameters are recorded by measuring light characteristics on the opposite side of the sphere with respect to the map or the terrain. When light characteristics change on the measured section by more than 25% per millisecond, it is necessary to profile an earthquake with magnitude 3 at the epicenter 14 days after the moment of recording. The earthquake epicenter is determined by scanning segments of the measured section. For the above case, light characteristics at the epicenter change by 32% per millisecond.

For production facilities, the functional diagram of the entire production process must be measured. When light characteristics at the measured section change by more than 14% per millisecond, it is necessary to profile deviations from the norm 14 days after the moment of recording. Detalization of the process that can have deviation from the norm is done by increasing the scale of the localized section of the diagram and taking the next measurement. In the element of the diagram that is the cause of deviations from the norm, light characteristics change by 32% per millisecond.

In the general case, schematizing any phenomenon of reality one can get a control forecast of events by measuring with this instrument the schemes corresponding to reality. Because when controlling an event a need can arise to create a substance with specified characteristics (for instance, emergency restoration of a microprocessor in a crashing aircraft) it is possible to specifically orient the instrument towards this process by placing the schematic of the substance above the third crystal of the module. The use of the mechanism for creating the required substance by applying principles contained in the crystal module makes it possible to create new environmentally safe industries. Calculation of instrument characteristics and measurement surfaces for some processes is done using a certain method, and in other processes a new method is developed for each process. In certain cases, when schematization of a phenomenon does not fully reflect the phenomenon parameters that are necessary for measurement (for instance, for fast-acting processes, microprocesses or some global catastrophes), irrational capabilities of determining the design data of the instrument are used. Because any phenomenon of reality, including an unknown one, can be described schematically, such instrument makes it possible to determine, and at the same time prevent, catastrophic processes from unknown fields of reality.

6. Optical Systems in the Control of Microprocesses

According to the theory of wave synthesis, control of microprocesses takes place in the area of synthesis. In microelectronics the application of fundamental definitions of optical systems takes place on a multicomponent basis. Each component can be defined by means of several parameters. Defining parameters of components can also be interrelated.

According to laws of quantum mechanics, in the elementary volume dтp of a pulse P-space of quantum states there is

$$dZ = 2\left(\frac{d\tau_p}{h^3}\right),$$

where

$$d\tau_p = dp_x \cdot dp_y \cdot dp_z \; ; \; h^3$$

is Planck's constant cubed.

Assuming that constant energy surfaces in P¬-space are presented by spheres, it is possible, based on the theory of wave synthesis, to control the number of quantum states N(E) using a method for converting a form of information corresponding to the effective mass of the electron near the bottom of the conduction band mn to the control pulse of the optical system. This technology can direct methods for the development and production of molecular devices toward complete environmental safety.

7. Conclusions

Based on the fundamental definitions of optical systems, data have been obtained for constructing an instrument for preventive forecast of catastrophes. The catastrophe forecast instrument built based on the analysis of light fluxes has functions of harmonic reduction or prevention of catastrophes. In such instrument, correction toward the maximum reduction of parameters of a catastrophe and the determination of characteristics of the phenomenon take place. According to the law of universal connections, such instrument-analytic structures pose no danger to humans or environment because they are realized based on safe characteristics of light. Using the control component of the optical system it is possible to create the required reality. The fundamental definitions of optical systems have the following expressions:

$$\Psi = \frac{E \cdot W}{U},$$

where Ψ is energy of the future, E is energy of the past, W is the space of distribution of energy of current time, and U is the space of distribution of energy of the past;

$$E = E_\text{н} \cdot F,$$

where E is energy of the present, and F is the function of intersection of energies of the future and the past;

$$W = \frac{\Psi \cdot W(1)}{E_\text{н}},$$

where W is common reality, and W1 is the function of common reality for fixable phenomena of any environment.

The novelty of definition of common reality is that for the first time the functional environment has

16

been defined that makes it possible to convert and describe any processes of reality from one point.

The field of application of the definition of common reality in optoconducting systems makes it possible to isolate the converting pulse of any environment and to control reality. In the general case, the discovery defines all phenomena of reality.

The effect of the fundamental definitions of optical systems is practical realization of laws of control optical pulse.

The first law is that crystal-based optical systems are reproducible as a reflection of future events after a picoseconds interval of the past.

The second law is the movement of an optical signal both in the direction of recording systems and into an environment of indefinable properties. As a result, it is possible to identify the information constant that determines control of environments with unknown structures.

The third law is that using the area of projection of the future onto the present as the basis of the pulse difference for various environments determines the structure of the instrument that harmonizes all systems.

The fourth law is that a system definable by an optical signal is always definable for processes of an infinite series. The corollary of the fourth law is that all processes of reality are described in each of its areas. The theory of wave synthesis has been derived. In describing reality, the theory of wave synthesis is formally expressed as follows:

$$T = Y \cdot S.$$

where T is time, Y is the wave of the dynamic phase of reality, and S is the stationary phase of reality. Studies of optical media in the direction of separation of optical pulse phases are conducted using the principle of minimizing the resistance of the medium along the pulse trajectory.

Applying the structure of the optical system derived in this work which makes it possible to harmonically forecast and prevent catastrophes, one can build instruments that, when used, do not cause any negative consequences in any time or space. A catastrophe that, by means of such instruments, is prevented or has reduced magnitude is already not realized anywhere. Equipment and any facilities that are created must be built using this harmonization principle. Such technology is safe for the producer and the environment. The crystal module for forecasting earthquakes is built based on such principle.

In the general case, schematizing any phenomenon of reality one can get a control forecast of events by measuring with this instrument the schemes corresponding to reality. For some reality processes (for instance, for fast-acting processes, microprocesses or some global catastrophes), instrument parameters are calculated by using sensory capabilities and taking into account understanding of laws of common connections. An irrational approach in calculating instrument parameters makes it possible to derive instrument functions from the analysis and definition of unknown properties of reality.

Appendix

Methods for Quantitative Calculation of a Module for Preventive Forecasting of Earthquakes and Catastrophes

Introduction

In order to have a quantitative calculation it is necessary to consider the entire operation process of the instrument and establish boundary and initial conditions for all intermediate cycles of the process. Dividing the problem into the process of light passage through the instrument and the process of measurement of output characteristics it is possible to find that one of the sources of acquiring output information is measurement of temperature in the area of the crystal. By using the theory of wave synthesis it turns out that in the calculations one can add the area of the dynamic wave of reality to the area of the static wave of reality, and from the area of reproduction of reality one can find the characteristics needed for measurement. In this particular case, labeling the radiation emitting from the area of measurement as the area of static reality S, one can use as the dynamic wave of reality Y laser radiation located on the side of the object of measurement and secured at the instrument. Then, in accordance with a fixed scale it will be possible to determine the time of an earthquake T taking into account the effect of laser radiation on the area of measurement of instrument parameters. According to the theory of wave synthesis, laser radiation amplifies informative parameters of sensed light radiation.

Orientation of the process of action of laser radiation on the structural material of a product must depend on characteristics of radiation from the measured object.

Studies of the action process are necessary first of all in order to substantiate structural materials used in a product and to issue recommendations for future development. The complexity of the research is due to the dependence of the character of the going process on thermophysical characteristics of the material and energy characteristics of laser radiation. For each specific case of laser radiation interaction with a material, a quite definitemathematil model of the process must be built that describes a real physical process, under assumptions that do not violate the model adequacy to the real physical process. Numerous original articles, reviews and monographs mainly present solutions of partial problems with a number of restrictions typical for a given model of interaction. This is why it became necessary to build mathematical models of interaction with specific materials. In my opinion, construction of a mathematical model that fairly accurately describes a physical process must be accompanied by experiments. Based on this, a computational-experimental method of solving problems was used, with digital simulation applied to it that makes it possible to convert objects of information to a geometric form.

Thus, the instrument is a crystal module, with the first crystal aimed toward the measured object, and with a thermocouple attached to the wall of the last crystal. Measurement of output characteristics via a thermocouple is one of the sources of information. The advantage of such source is higher noise immunity.

The use of laser radiation by applying the theory of wave synthesis also solves the problem of stability of the signal emitted from the measured objects. Because radiation emitted from an object for the version of measurement of characteristics via a thermocouple is a partial problem of the process of laser radiation, it is clear that the main thing is the calculation of the process of laser radiation.

1. Interaction of Continuous Laser Radiation With Materials

1.1 Heat Transmission in a Homogeneous Layer of Substance

The thermal state of an illuminated material and the character of physical processes are determined by electric characteristics of laser radiation – flux density and time of action of laser radiation, the space distribution of intensity in the beam, and by geometric parameters and thermophysical characteristics of the illuminated material.

Energy of laser radiation E concentrated on the surface of the illuminated material is distributed as follows:

$$E = E_{OTP} + E_{\Pi O\Gamma\Pi} + E_{\Pi P O\Pi,}$$

where E_{OTP} is energy mirror-like and diffusely reflected by the illuminated surface; $E_{\Pi O\Gamma\Pi}$ is energy of laser radiation absorbed by the material; and $E_{\Pi P O\Pi}$ is energy of laser radiation passed through the material (for transparent materials). Only the absorbed portion of energy was taken into account.

In the work, heating of materials is calculated using the classic theory of thermal conductivity.

The basis of this approach is that light energy instantly converts to heat at the point where light has been absorbed. Energy is distributed so fast that local equilibrium exists during the entire time of laser radiation action. Therefore, one can use the concept of temperature and regular equations for heat flow. In practically interesting cases we can consider this a one-dimensional problem. This is possible when cross-sectional dimensions of a laser beam are large compared to the depth of heat propagation during the time of action of laser radiation and when for calculation of heat transmission in other directions one can use the model of heat transmission in a heterogeneous layer of substance; this model is described later. To clarify the characteristics of space distribution of radiation one can use the principle of integration of distributed temperatures; however, this is not necessary because by using the theory of wave synthesis it is possible to get the necessary number of clarifications at any point of the process using the specified in the introduction method of the static and dynamic phases of reality based on fundamental discoveries of optical systems. We will assume that the distribution of intensity of laser radiation in a beam is uniform and cylindrical. We will assume that absorption factor of laser radiation A is temperature-dependent. The differential equation describing heat transmission in a homogeneous layer of substance has the following form:

$$\frac{\partial T}{\partial \tau} = a \cdot \frac{\partial^2 T}{\partial x^2} \qquad (1)$$
$$0 \leq x \leq l,$$
$$0 \leq \tau < \infty,$$

where T is temperature; τ is time; x is space;

$$a \cdot \frac{k}{C \cdot \rho}$$

is thermal diffusivity; k is coefficient of thermal conductivity; C is specific heat; ρ is density; and l is the

20

thickness of the layer of substance.

The initial condition is:

$$T|_{x=0} = T_0. \qquad (2)$$

The boundary condition on the illuminated surface is:

$$K\frac{\partial T}{\partial x}\bigg|_{x=0} = \varepsilon b\left(T_\pi^4 - T_c^4\right) + \alpha(t_\pi - t_c) - \qquad (3)$$
$$- \rho \cdot A_\lambda(T),$$

ε is emissivity; b is the Stefan-Boltzmann constant; T_π is absolute temperature of the body surface; T_C is absolute temperature of the environment;

$$a = \frac{Nu \cdot \lambda}{l_1}$$

is heat exchange coefficient,

where Nu is the Nusselt number; λ is coefficient of thermal conductivity of the cooling medium; l_1 is characteristic dimension of the unit area; t_π is surface temperature of the body; and T_C is temperature of the cooling medium.

$$Nu = 0{,}57 \cdot R_l^{0,5}$$

in the case of laminar flow of the cooling medium; and

$$Nu = 0{,}32 \cdot R_l^{0,8}$$

in the case of turbulent flow of the cooling medium.

$$R_l = \frac{v \cdot l_1}{v}$$

is the Reynolds number (at $R_i < 5 \cdot 10^5$ flow of the cooling medium will be laminar),

where v is kinematic viscosity of the cooling medium, and ρ is flux density of laser radiation.

The boundary condition on the back surface is:

$$K\frac{\partial T}{\partial x}\bigg|_{x=1} = -\varepsilon b\left(T_\pi^4 - T_c^4\right) + \alpha(t_\pi - t_c). \qquad (4)$$

The boundary condition when there is heat insulation on the back surface is:

$$K \frac{\partial T}{\partial x}\bigg|_{x=l} = 0. \qquad (4^*)$$

The system consisting of differential heat transfer equation (1), initial condition (2) and boundary conditions (3) and (4) or (4*) is a mathematical model of the process of laser radiation interaction with material. Such nonlinear problem poses considerable difficulties even for a solution using numerical methods because summands containing temperatures to the fourth degree strongly affect stability of difference schemes, and control of the scheme convergence requires much longer computing time. For numerical solution of the problem let us use the method of networks per explicit 1st order difference scheme (В области = "In area")

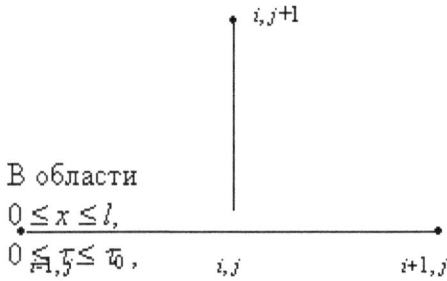

В области
$0 \le x \le l,$
$0 \le \tau \le \tau_0,$

$i,j+1$
i,j
$i+1,j$

where τ0 is the time of material exposure to laser radiation, and let us introduce the following network:

$$x_i = i \cdot h; i = 0 \div M; h = \frac{l}{M};$$

$$\tau_j = j \cdot \Delta \tau, j = 0 \div N; \Delta \tau = \frac{\tau_0}{N};$$

22

Where h is an increment of space coordinate; $\Delta\tau$ is an increment of time interval; M is the number of nodes of space breakdown; and N is the number of nodes of time breakdown.

Then finite difference approximation of equation (1) is written in the following form:

$$\frac{T_{i,j+1} - T_{i,j}}{\Delta\tau} = a\,\frac{T_{i+1,j} - 2T_{i,j} + T_{i-1,j}}{h^2}$$

Let

$$\omega = \Delta\tau \cdot \frac{a}{h^2},$$

Then

$$T_{i,j+1} = (1 - 2\cdot\omega)T_{i,j} + \omega\cdot(T_{i+1,j} + T_{i-1,j}). \qquad (5)$$

Finite difference approximation of equation (2) has the following form:

$$T_{i,0} = T_0. \qquad (6)$$

Finite difference approximation of equation (3) is written in the following form:

$$T = T_{1,J+1} - Q_1 T_{1,J} + Q_2 T_{1,J} + Q_3 T_{2,J} + Q_0 + Q \qquad (7)$$

where

$$Q_1 = G\cdot\left(\frac{k}{h} + \frac{Nu\cdot\lambda}{l_1}\right); \quad Q_2 = G\cdot\varepsilon\cdot b;$$

$$Q_3 = G\,k/h, Q = G\left(\varepsilon\cdot b\cdot T_0^4 + \frac{Nu\cdot\lambda}{l_1}\cdot T_0\right);$$

$$Q_0 = \rho\cdot A(T)\cdot G;\ G = 2\cdot\Delta\tau/k\cdot h.$$

Finite difference approximation of equation (4) has the following form:

$$T_{M,j+1} = T_{M,j} + Q_1\cdot T_{M,j} + Q_2\cdot T^*_{M\,j} -$$
$$- Q_3\cdot T_{M-1,j} - Q, \qquad (8)$$

and for equation (4*)

$$T_{M,j+1} = T_{M,j} + \frac{2 \cdot \Delta \tau}{h^2}\left(T_{M-1,j} - T_{M,j}\right). \quad (8^*)$$

Convergence of the constructed difference scheme can be ensured by varying ω. In doing this it is necessary to find the optimum, from the standpoint of saving computing time, value of ω that ensures convergence of this difference scheme. It is desirable to determine the value of ω for each specific case, depending on the material thickness, time of exposure to laser radiation and thermophysical properties of materials.

1.2 Heat Transmission in a Heterogeneous Layer of Substance

In the instrument, the intermediate medium between the crystals determines expansion of the calculation procedure to multilayer materials characterized by heterogeneity along different directions. A schematic of such materials is shown in Fig. 1.

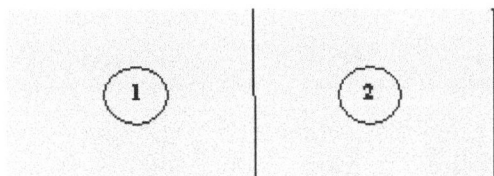

Fig. 1

The differential equation describing heat transmission process
In layer 1 has the following form:

$$\frac{\partial T_1}{\partial \tau} = a_1 \cdot \frac{\partial^2 T_1}{\partial x^2},$$
$$0 \leq x \leq l,$$
$$0 \leq t < \infty.$$

For layer 2

$$\frac{\partial T_2}{\partial \tau} = a_2 \cdot \frac{\partial^2 T_2}{\partial x^2},$$
$$l < x \leq L,$$
$$0 \leq \tau < \infty.$$

The initial conditions:

24

$$T_1|_{\tau=0} = T_1^0 \,;$$
$$T_2|_{\tau=0} = T_2^0 \,.$$

The boundary conditions at the illuminated and back surface of the material are similar to boundary conditions in Section 1.1. The boundary conditions in the area of layers interface, under the condition of an ideal heat contact, have the following form:

$$T_1|_{x=0} = T_2|_{x=0} \,, \qquad (11)$$

$$K_1 \frac{\partial T_1}{\partial x}\bigg|_{x=1} = K_2 \cdot \frac{\partial T_2}{\partial x}\bigg|_{x=1} \qquad (12)$$

The finite difference approximation of equation (11) is

$$T_{1_{i,j}} = T_{2_{i,j}} \,. \qquad (14)$$

The finite difference approximation of equation (12) is

$$T_{1_{i,j+1}} = Q_4 \cdot T_{1_{i-1,j}} + Q_5 \cdot T_{1_{i,j}} - Q_9 \cdot T_{2_{i+1,j}} \,, \qquad (15)$$

where

$$Q_4 = \frac{K_1}{K_2 - K_1} \cdot \frac{\Delta \tau}{h^2} \,;$$

$$Q_5 = (h^2 - \Delta \tau) \cdot K_2 - (h^2 + \Delta \tau) \cdot K_1 \,;$$

$$Q_9 = \frac{K_2}{K_2 - K_1} \cdot \frac{\Delta \tau}{h^2} \,.$$

It is easy to transfer the derived result to a multilayer model of material.

Cyclic calculations based on the derived finite difference formulae describe the process of non-stationary heat conduction in a material. First, in accordance with initial conditions, one makes an initial assignment:

$$T_n|_{\tau=0} = T_n^0, \, N = 1, 2 \dots,$$

where N is the number of layers of the material.

In addition, one should take into account dependence of the absorption factor on the surface temperature. The absorption factor will be determined in accordance with experimental data. The constructed mathematical model is applicable before a material begins melting.

2. Effect of Pulse-Periodic Laser Radiation on Structural Materials

To increase the instrument life and reduce the requirements to surface finish of the crystals one can use pulse-periodic laser radiation.

When constructing a mathematical model of the process of interaction of pulse-periodic laser radiation with a material it is necessary first of all consider the possibility of replacing pulse-periodic radiation with quasi-continuous radiation.

Let τ_l be the interval between the pulses, τ_0 the pulse length, and $\tau_n = \tau_0 + \tau_l$ is the pulse repetition period.

If τ is the time of action of radiation, then the conditions for the replacement with quasi-continuous radiation have the following form:

$$\bar{\tau}_n \ll \sqrt{\tau_0 \tau}. \qquad (16)$$

If condition (16) is not satisfied, i.e., if the quasi-continuous process of laser radiation action on a material does not approximate, then one considers the determinacy of components of the pulse-periodic process. At the initial time moment after pulse action has stopped, an isotherm with fixed temperature moves deep inside the material and then, after reaching certain depth, the isotherm moves back. The isotherm position by the start of the next pulse makes it possible to determine the depth of material heating. Thus, the solution derived for continuous action of laser radiation is generalized to the case of pulse-periodic character of laser radiation where pulse length τ_0 is used as the time of action.

In cyclic calculations during quantitative realization of finite difference equations the cool-down mode is specified by deleting the term $\rho \cdot A(\tau) \cdot S(Q_0)$ from equation (7) for the duration time τ_l (corresponding to the interval between pulses), and the set of temperatures obtained after time τ_l elapses is considered the initial set for the heating mode. The heating mode is specified by including term Q_0 for the duration of the time of action for pulse τ_0.

When describing the action of millisecond laser pulses with radiation flux density of up to 10 W/cm2 on optical surfaces it is necessary to take into account that:

-energy losses on reradiation and due to convection from the heated surface can be take into account by using a model of a conditional moving boundary of the absorbing surface; and

- the thermophysical formulation of the problem in accordance with the theory of wave synthesis that describes laser radiation interaction with the source radiation and a material is only valid for flux densities that do no cause changing of optical characteristics of the instrument before the end of its operating life.

3. Conducting Experimental Work

The results of experimental work conducted using the experimental unit were used for correcting conversion factors for converting objects of information to geometric forms. Then, functional parameters of the forms were established, and simulation aimed at forecasting real earthquakes was performed. Output infor-

26

mation can be measured via a thermocouple, indicator of optical signals, etc.

The goal of conducting experimental work on the experimental unit is to find the dependence of temperature of the back surface of the illuminated specimen of a material on the time of action of laser radiation with specified density ρ.

The results of experimental work conducted using the experimental unit were used for correcting conversion factors for converting objects of information to geometric forms. Then, functional parameters of the forms were established, and simulation aimed at forecasting real earthquakes was performed. Output information can be measured via a thermocouple, indicator of optical signals, etc.

The goal of conducting experimental work on the experimental unit is to find the dependence of temperature of the back surface of the illuminated specimen of a material on the time of action of laser radiation with specified density ρ.

The following experimental equipment was used:

1.　　Heat treatment unit 02TL-3600-004 (the experimental unit – ЭУ).

2.　　Thermocouple type TT-243 (sensor – Д).

3.　　Extension thermoelectrode wires, copper-titanium-nickel-copper type (МТ-НИ).

4.　　Digital millivoltmeter щ-300 (information presentation device – СПИ).

The block diagram of the experimental work is presented in Fig 2:

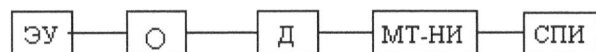

Fig. 2

O – specimen of the studied material

A schematic diagram of the experimental unit with a studied specimen and measurement means is presented in Fig. 3.

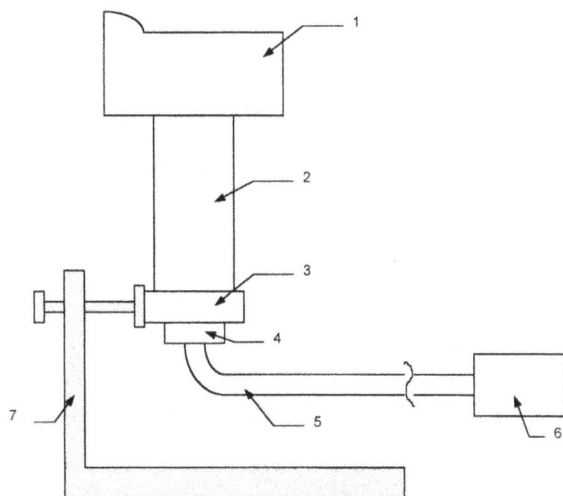

Fig. 3

1 – ЭУ; 2 – beam; 3 – material specimen; 4 – sensor; 5 – thermoelectrode wires; 6 – voltmeter; 7 – clamp for securing the material specimen

In the unite 1, a laser beam 2 with certain flux density ρ is generated. On its way the beam 2 encounters a material specimen 3 secured on the clamp 7. A thermocouple 5 is attached to the specimen back surface. Thermoelectrode wires 6 go from the thermocouple 5 to the voltmeter (7) *[sic]*. Voltmeter readings are recorded after certain time intervals. Then, using a special table the readings are converted to temperatures that correspond to temperatures at those time moments.

Main sources of errors when measuring temperature are disturbances of homogeneity of the material layer due to the introduction of thermoelectronic converter into it, as well as removal of heat over the converter wires. The character of testing the temperature field when making a slot for placing a temperature sensor is shown in Fig. 4a and 4б.

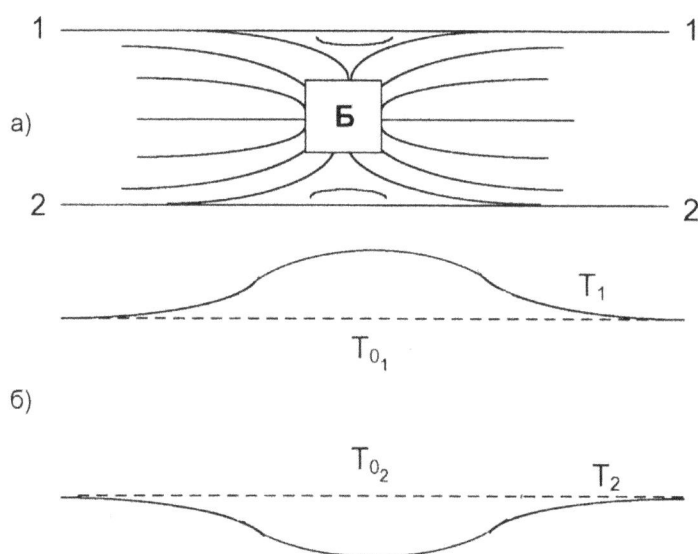

Fig. 4

a – isotherms; б – temperature on surfaces 1-1 and 2-2

It is practically impossible to determine the exact place where the thermoelectric sensor junction touches the slot surface; because of this, there is uncertainty when measuring temperature in the interval $dT = T_A - T_Б$. The total measurement error was 4%.

Graphs of time dependence of temperature of the back surface were plotted as follows:

1)   results obtained in cases of gross measurement errors were excluded, as invalid, from the results of a series of experiments conducted under equivalent conditions;

2) the remaining results, i.e., the results of experiments where the measurement error pertain to the class of systematic errors, was used to plot families of curves that express temperature dependence of the back surface of the material;

3) for each family of curves corresponding to each specific case, the average curve that characterizes time

28

dependence of temperature was determined.

After obtaining a graph of dependence of temperature of a specimen back surface on time, numerical calculation of the problem of the inverse mathematical model was performed. If experimental results differed from the results of numerical calculation by more than 9%, the value of the absorption factor was corrected. This is how it is possible to find temperature dependence of absorption factor A for each studied material. The use of temperature dependences of absorption factors makes it possible to determine temperature fields of studied materials with sufficient for engineering calculation accuracy (up to 9%) while using only a mathematical module. When describing the process of laser radiation interaction with structural materials in vacuum the mathematical model is simplified because term $a(t_n - t_c)$ which characterizes convective heat exchange is excluded from equation (3).

For preventive forecast of earthquakes, the source of radiation is a map of the terrain. For preventive forecast of catastrophes at industrial facilities, the source of radiation is the schematic diagram of the industrial facility that includes description of production cycles (in this case, the instrument records changes in the specific section of the diagram). The instrument action can be applied to any objects of reality, including objects with unknown properties. To do this, it is necessary to use the coefficient of thermal conductivity of the static phase of reality and the coefficient of emissivity of the dynamic phase.

Conclusion

1.	Using the theory of wave synthesis and fundamental discoveries of optical systems, a computational-experimental method for solving nonlinear problems of action of continuous or pulse-periodic action of laser radiation for preventive forecast of earthquakes and catastrophes of industrial facilities and for forecast-oriented control of microprocesses has been constructed and substantiated. The solution is applicable to cases of any catastrophe, including catastrophes from environments with unknown properties.

2.	Formulas (5), (6), (7), (8), (8*), (14) and (15) have been derived in a final form which make it possible to realize the constructed mathematical model numerically.
Shown are the algorithm for calculation of temperature fields based on the derived finite difference formulae and ways for optimizing the algorithm from the standpoint of saving computing time.

Results of using the theory of wave synthesis and fundamental discoveries of optical systems have been obtained which make it possible to describe, with accuracy sufficient for engineering calculations, the real physical process both in gaseous medium and in vacuum.

29

References

1.	Grabovoi, G.P., "Прикладные структуры создающей области информации" ["Applied Structures of the Creating Information Field"], Moscow, Kalashnikov Publishing House, 1998.

2.	Certificates-Licenses of the International Chamber of Registration of Information and Intellectual Novelty issued to Grigori Grabovoi for sections Discoveries, Principle, Method, and Model. Registration numbers: 000287, 000284, 000286, 000285. 000283. Date of issue: December 19, 1997.

Scientific and Technical Collection "ELECTRONIC TECHNOLOGY", series 3
"MICROELECTRONICS", Volume 1 (153), 1999, Central Scientific Research Institute "Elektronika",
Moscow.
Article by Grigori Grabovoi "Studies and Analysis of the Basic Definitions".

3.	Grabovoi, G.P, "Практика управления. Путь спасения" ["The Practice of Management. The Road to Salvation"], Vol. 1-3, Moscow "Soprichastnost" Publishing House, 1998.

4.	Grabovoi, G.P., "Унифицированная система знаний" ["The Unified Knowledge System"], Moscow, Kalshnikov Publishing House, 1996.

5.	Decision of granting a patent to Grigori Grabovoi for the invention on the method for prevention of catastrophes and a device for implementation thereof. Rospatent, No. 99120836/28 of January 28, 2000.

Received December 11, 1999

Electronic Technology. Series 3. Microelctronics. Vol. 1 (153), 1999

The "Science Center" Graduate School

**is announcing the opening of a new Department "Forecast-Oriented Quality
Systems of the Development and Manufacturing of Microelectronics Products,
Their Marketing, Management and Financial Support".
Department Science Adviser - Grigori Grabovoi.
For information call 530 98 30.**

31

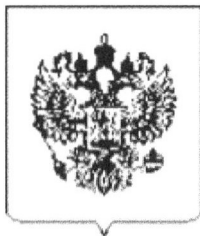

(19) RU (11) 2148845 (13) C1

(51) 7 G01V9/00 G01V8/20

**FEDERAL SERVICE
FOR INTELLECTUAL PROPERTY,
PATENTS AND TRADEMARKS
(ROSPATENT)**

(12) DESCRIPTION OF THE PATENT
of the Russian Federation

(14) Publication date: **05.10.2000**
(21) Application registration number: **99120836/28**
(22)   Filing date: **10.07.1999**
(24) Date of patent: **10.07.1999**
(46) Date of publication of the claims: **05.10.2000**
(56) Analogs of the invention: **RU 2107933 C1, 03.27.1998
RU 2050014 C1, 12.10.1995. RU 2098850 C1,
12.10.1997. SU 1104459 A, 07.23.1984.**

(71) Applicant: **Grabovoi Grigori
Petrovich (aka Grigori Grabovoi®)**
(72) Inventor: **Grigori Grabovoi®**
(73) Patentee: **Grigori Grabovoi®**
(98) Address for correspondence: **115230,
Moscow, Kashirskoe Shosse
5-1-66, Kopaev, V.G.**

(54) A METHOD FOR PREVENTION OF CATASTROPHES AND A DEVICE FOR IMPLEMENTATION THEREOF

The use: for prevention of natural or anthropogenic catastrophes. The essence: light radiation signals from a component corresponding to the zone of the anticipated catastrophe are processed using an optical system comprising sensory elements made from a crystal, for instance, from rock crystal, that have the shape of identical cubes arranged along the direction of propagation of the radiation and placed in a glass sphere. The last cube is connected by means of an optical fiber to a transducer; the transducer is connected via an amplifier to a processor system. In the optical system, normalized radiation is formed. It is preferable to conduct scanning of various sections of a component made, for instance, in the form of a terrain map, wherein the zone with increased parameters of normalized radiation corresponds to the section of the origination of the catastrophe. Thus, for natural catastrophes, the section of the origination of the catastrophe has characteristics that are 20-28% higher than characteristics of radiation from other sections of the component, and for anthropogenic catastrophes the respective increase is 10-12%. The technical result: increased efficiency while at the same time expanding the fields of application of the claimed method and device.

ɔject is achieved by the new method for prevention of catastrophes by timely forecasting an incipient
ɔphe and generating signals that normalize the situation in the zone of the anticipated catastrophe,
thod being implemented by means of the new device.

According to the invention, the method for prevention of catastrophes is implemented by recor-
ıd processing signals characterizing the situation in the zone of the anticipated catastrophe, wher-
nals of light radiation from a component corresponding to the zone of the anticipated catastrophe
ıcessed using an optical system comprising sensory elements made of aligned crystals arranged in
ı along the direction of the sensed radiation, and normalized radiation is formed in the system in
ɔ normalize the situation in the zone of the anticipated catastrophe; and it is preferable to: conduct
ıous scanning of various sections of the component corresponding to the zone of the anticipated
ɔphe, identifying the section of the origination of the catastrophe by the increase of characteristics
ation coming out of the optical system compared to characteristics of radiation from other sections;
y sections of origination of a natural catastrophe by a 20-28% increase of characteristics of radiation
ɔonding to this section compared to characteristics of radiation from two sections; define the section
ɔrigination of an anthropogenic catastrophe by a 10 -12% increase of characteristics of radiation cor-
ding to this section compared to characteristics of radiation from other sections.

ling to the invention, the device for prevention of catastrophes comprises a converter of signals cha-
ıing the situation in the zone of the anticipated catastrophe, a system for recording the signals, and a
ır that generates signals facilitating normalization in the zone, wherein the signal converter comprises
ɔonent corresponding to the zone of the anticipated catastrophe, and an optical system comprising:
y elements made of aligned crystals arranged in tandem along the direction of the sensed light ra-
. that have the shape of identical cubes shifted with respect to each other and having different ori-
ns of their optical axes wherein respective planes of the cubes are parallel; a glass sphere the cubes
ated in and form a continuous transparent structure with; and a transducer of normalized radiation
ted by means of an optical fiber to the last cube in the direction of radiation propagation and connec-
ı processor system; and it is preferable to: make the signal transducer in the form of a combination of
ical system and a terrain map where a catastrophic earthquake is anticipated to originate; make the
transducer in the form of a combination of the optical system and a telemetry system with a monitor
the component corresponding to the zone of anticipated anthropogenic catastrophe is displayed; to
e the processor system program package with all kinds of parameters of zones of anticipated catast-
.

The invention is based on the theory of wave synthesis developed by the applicant, combined with
ımula of general reality (see the thesis for the degree of a Doctor of Physical and Mathematical Sci-
Grigori Grabovoi, "Исследование и анализ фундаментальных определений оптических систем
ɔогноза землетрясений и катастроф производственных объектов" [Research and Analysis of
Definitions of Optical Systems for Forecasting Earthquakes and Catastrophes of Industrial Facilities],
w, RAEN Publishing House, 1999, pp. 9 - 19). According to the theory of wave synthesis, reality can
ved as a periodic intersection of stationary and dynamic regions, wherein the synthesis of a dynamic
ınd a stationary wave occurs in the intersection zones. In crystals, a similar process makes it possible,

DESCRIPTION OF THE INVENTION

The invention can be used for prevention of various catastrophic phenomena, w
instance, catastrophic earthquakes, or anthropogenic catastrophic phenomena, particula
facilities.

The closest to the claimed method in the technical essence is the method for pre
catastrophe – an earthquake – by recording and processing signals that characterize the
of the anticipated catastrophe (see the USSR certificate of authorship No. 1030496, cl.]
According to the known method, vibration signals in the form of vibration of Earth's cr
earthquake epicenter are processed using a network of geophones by receiving electric
tion acquisition, recording and processing centers the received signals are converted to
fed to radiators made in the form of vibration sources. The generated or normalized sig
elastic wave oscillations are sent to the earthquake origination zone. Seismic vibrations
interaction of high-frequency elastic vibrations from the vibration sources with low-fre
tions from the earthquake epicenter.

The shortcoming of the known method is its low efficiency because a counterac
earthquake is only conducted when the earthquake has reached sufficient degree of dev
of this it is necessary first to receive a number of predictive signals at the information a
and processing center. Besides, the known method has limited functional capabilities be
used for preventing earthquakes and is useless for preventing other catastrophic phenon
anthropogenic catastrophes.

The closest to the claimed device in the technical essence is the device for preve
catastrophe – an earthquake - comprising a converter of signals that characterize the loc
of the anticipated catastrophe, and a radiator that generates signals facilitating normaliz
tion in the zone of the anticipated catastrophe (see USSR Certificate of Authorship No.
31/08, 1981). The known device uses as the signal converter a vibration transducer that
cal vibrations originating during an earthquake to electric signals the amplitude of whic
the amplitude of mechanical vibrations. The signal processing system comprises a prea
for separation of basic frequency, a module for automatic phase tracking where the pha
shifted 180°, and a power amplifier. The radiator is made in the form of a vibration com
vibrations that have the phase opposite to the phase of vibrations generated during an e
facilitate normalization of the situation in the zone of origination of the earthquake.

The shortcomings of the known device are its limited functional capabilities bec
be used when there is a catastrophic earthquake. Besides, the operation of the known de
expense due to unusually high power consumption because of the need to radiate mecha
sufficiently long time.

The object of the invention is to increase the efficiency of the method for preven
while at the same time expanding functional capabilities of the claimed method and the
implementation thereof, and to reduce the cost of implementation of the method.

Said
catas
the m

ding
ein si
are p
tande
order
conti
catas
of rac
identi
corre
of the
respo
Acco
racter
radiat
a com
senso
diatio
entati
are lo
conne
ted to
the op
signa
where
provi
rophe

the fc
ences
для п
Basic
Mosc
be vie
wave

by solving the inverse problem, to derive from a stationary medium in the form of a crystal the dynamic components of wave synthesis, i.e., the time phase. With certain arrangements of crystals in space, the medium that is the source of a certain component of light normalizes. Thus, it becomes possible to normalize the medium the information about which is contained in the light component. Besides, it is possible to

the time of deviation from the norm after the optical system resources are exhausted, for instance, to determine the time of the earthquake or catastrophe. Normalization of the situation in the zone of the anticipated catastrophe is facilitated by the use of the radiator in the form of a microprocessor; normalization of the situation in the zone of the anticipated catastrophe is accomplished by means of the optical system that receives information from the radiating medium; the system is comprised of aligned crystals arranged in tandem along the direction of the sensed light radiation. As a radiating medium one can use a terrain map or a telemetry system with a monitor. When light from the radiating medium arrives at sensory elements of the optical system, the initial action of normalizing the radiating medium by the first crystal occurs at the moment when the component of light from the third crystal passes through the fourth crystal, and the next normalizing action occurs when the component of light passes through all the crystals. Light has been selected as the information-carrying medium because this will make it possible to visualize and record the laws of relations established by the formula of general reality. As the source for receiving output information one can use a normalized radiation transducer made, for instance, in the form of a temperature transducer connected to the last sensory element. Signals from the transducer are recorded using a processor system the transducer and radiator are connected to. The use of the program package with all kinds of parameters of zones of anticipated catastrophes makes it possible to increase the efficiency of the claimed device. In the general case, the claimed method and device make it possible to convert, for decrease or prevention, information, in the form of light pulses, about both natural and anthropogenic catastrophes, and forecasting and prevention of all kinds of catastrophic phenomena can be performed from any point in space.

The attached drawings show the following: Fig. 1 shows the arrangement of sensory elements in the optical system (projection on plane OX, O2, where OX is the horizontal direction and O2 is the vertical direction), Fig. 2 shows the general view of the device used for implementation of the method for prevention of catastrophes, and Fig. 3 shows the general view of the device used for implementation of the method for prevention of catastrophes.

The device comprises: sensory elements 1, 2, 3, 4, 5, 6, and 7 in the form of identical size cubes that are located in the glass sphere 8 and form a transparent monolithic system with it; an optical fiber 9 that connects the last sensory element with the normalized radiation transducer 10; a laser 11; a component 12 corresponding to the zone of the anticipated catastrophe made, for instance, in the form of a terrain map; ан amplifier 13 of signals from the transducer, the amplifier installed at the input of a processor system 14 that has a package of programs for processing signals from the transducer and is connected to a display 15 and to a radiator 16 of signals facilitating normalization of the situation in the zone of the anticipated catastrophe; and an object 17 generating bioelectric signals.

The number of sensory elements in the optical system can be set at 7, 14, etc. Sensory elements 1-7 are made from crystals, for instance, from rock crystal or diamonds, in the form of identical size cubes that, for instance, have the face length of 20 mm. When the material of the glass sphere 8 secures the cubes, the side faces of all cubes are positioned parallel to each other. The arrangement of cubes 1 - 7 in the sphere 8 and orientation of their optical axes are selected such that prevention of catastrophic phenomena, for instance, earthquakes, with harmonization occurs. The cubes are shifted with respect to each other in two mutually perpendicular planes as shown in Fig. 1 and Fig. 2. The output parameters of the optical system are recorded using the normalized radiation transducer 10 located on the side of the sphere 8 opposite to the terrain map 12. It is preferable to make the transducer 20 in the form of a fast-response supersensitive film component serving, for instance, as a temperature transducer. The use of the laser 11 makes it possible to increase the accuracy of measurement of signals from the transducer 10. The use of the object that generates bioelectric signals additionally facilitates normalization of the situation in the zone of the anticipated catastrophe. The operation of the device is described when describing the claimed method for prevention of catastrophes.

According to the claimed method, light radiation from the component 12 corresponding to the zone of the anticipated catastrophe, which is made, for instance, in the form of a full-scale terrain map is aimed at the optical system comprising the glass sphere 8 wherein sensory elements 1-7 made of aligned crystals arranged in tandem along the direction of the sensed light radiation are located. When converting light radiation in such optical system (see Fig. 3), a normalized to the maximum light volume is released. Normalization occurs when a light component passes through sensory elements 1-7; their mutual arrangement causes harmonization of the light volume which in turn normalizes the situation in the zone of the anticipated catastrophe. Herein, the degree of alleviation of the catastrophic phenomenon is commensurate with the amount of normalization of the light volume. After passing through the amplifier 13, signals from the normalized radiation transducer 10 are transmitted to the processor system 14 containing a package of programs for processing of incoming signals. After the signals are processed, their characteristics are displayed on display 5. When a catastrophic phenomenon is forecast, radiator 16 is activated, and additional signals which facilitate normalization of the situation in this zone are sent to the zone of the anticipated catastrophe. It is preferable to conduct continuous scanning of various sections of the component 12 corresponding to the zone of the anticipated catastrophe by means of sequential absorption of radiation coming from the component 12 in all sensory elements 1-7. Herein, the section of the origination of the catastrophe is identified by the increase of characteristics of radiation from this section compared to characteristics of radiation from other sections. During the origination of a natural catastrophe, for instance, of an earthquake, characteristics of radiation from the section of the origination of the catastrophe are 20 - 28% higher than the characteristics of other sections of the component 12. When characteristics of radiation increase by less than 20%, catastrophic phenomenon will occur, and when characteristics of radiation increase by more than 28%, one can conclude that an emergency catastrophic phenomenon is developing. During origination of an anthropogenic catastrophe, for instance, of a catastrophe related to failure of a nuclear reactor work cycle, the section of the origination of the catastrophe is identified by a 10-12% increase of characteristics of radiation. When characteristics of radiation increase by less than 10%, no catastrophic phenomenon will occur, and when characteristics of radiation increase by more than 12%, one can

36

expect an extreme course of events.

Below are examples of implementation of the claimed method using a prototype of the claimed device comprising an optical system consisting of a glass sphere wherein seven sensory elements made of rock crystal in the form of identical size cubes with the face length of 20 mm are distributed in tandem. The normalized

Radiation

$\downarrow$

Излучение
$\longrightarrow$

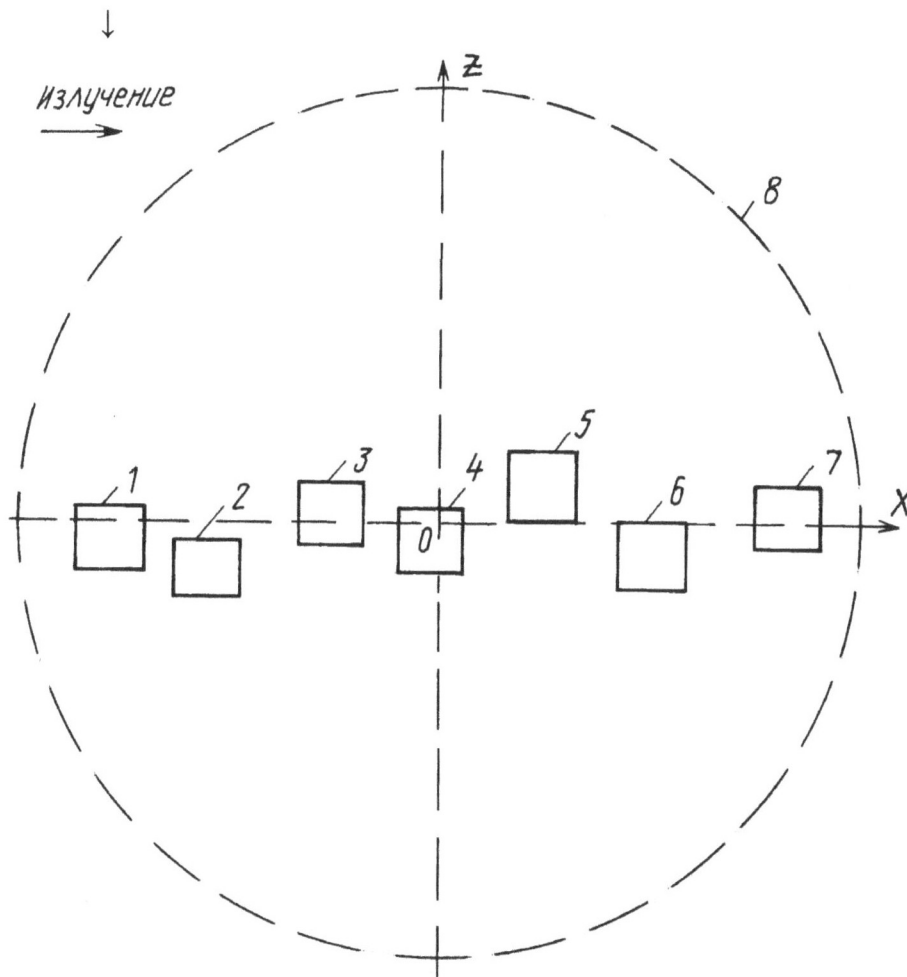

Фиг. 1

Fig. 1 ↑

Radiation
↓

Излучение →

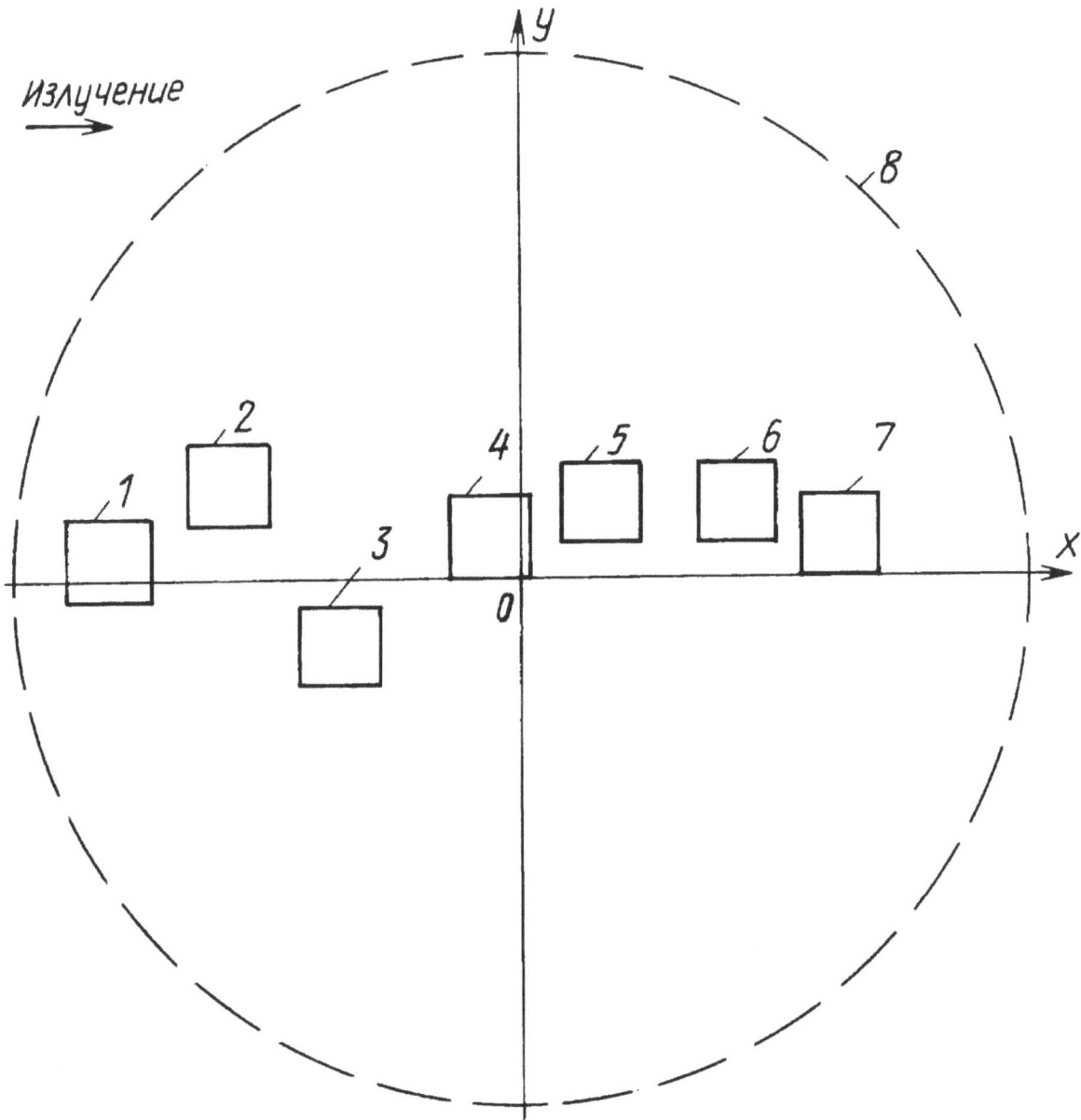

Фиг. 2

↑
Fig. 2

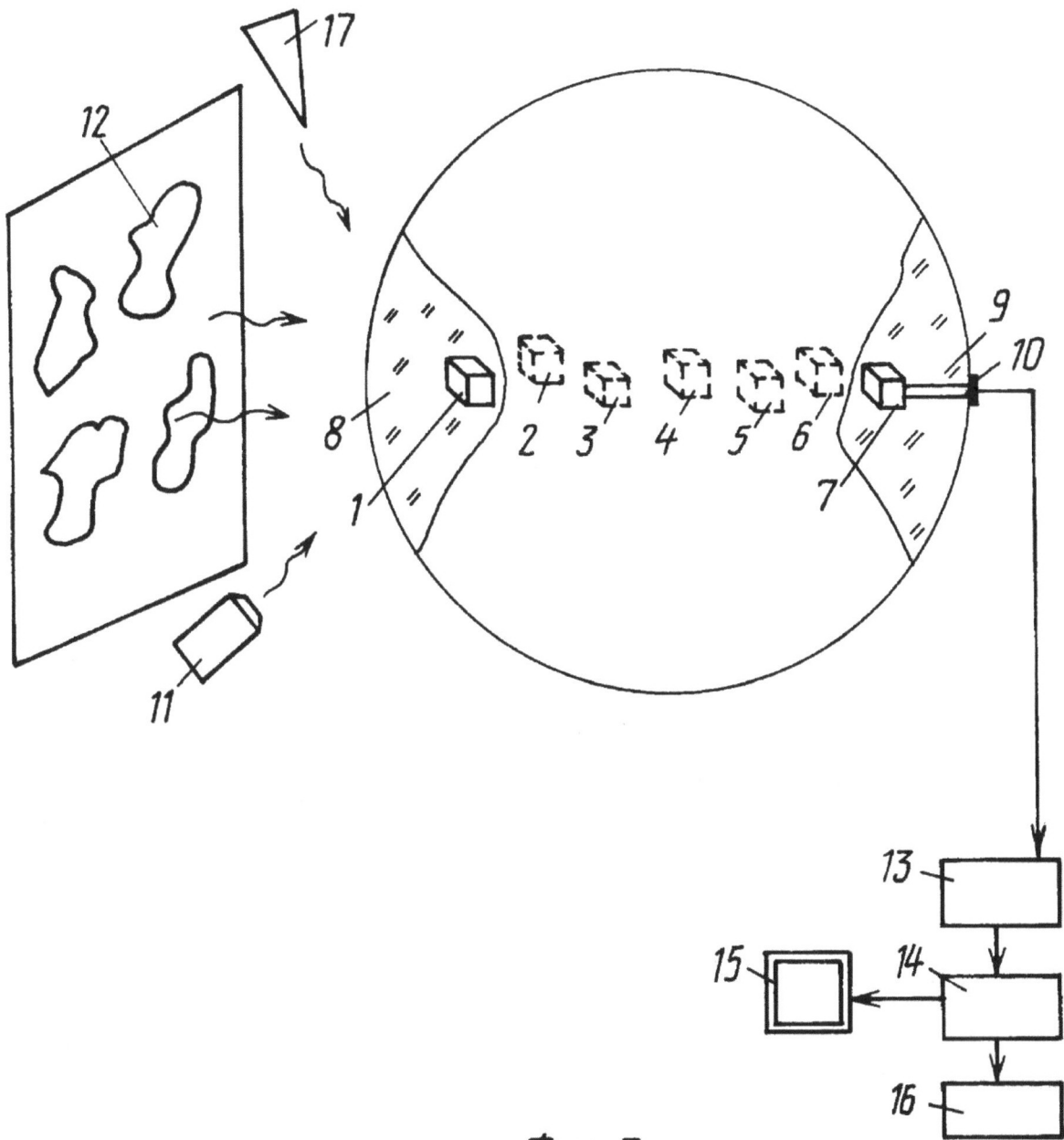

Фиг. 3

↑
Fig. 3

radiation transducer in the form of a thin-film temperature transducer is connected by means of an optical fiber to the last cube in the direction of propagation of light radiation. The transducer is connected via the amplifier to the processor system input made with the capability of accelerated calculation of a quadruple integrator.

Example 1. The origination of a catastrophic earthquake in the Kamchatka region was studied. The glass sphere 8 with sensory elements 1-7 was placed at a distance of 250 mm from a full-scale map of Kamchatka; the normalized radiation transducer 10 was placed on the side of the sphere 8 opposite the side facing the map. Signals from the transducer 10 were passing through the amplifier 13 and entering the processor system 14 where they were continuously processed, recorded and displayed on the display 15. Measurements were taken during a period beginning at 09:03 on June 26 1999. The origination of a 5.1 magnitude earthquake had been forecast; it happened at 09:03 on July 03, 1999, and due to the use of the claimed device its magnitude decreased by 0.4 points.

Example 2. Under the same conditions as in the example above, scanning of the component 12 corresponding to the zone of anticipated earthquake – a map of Japan - was conducted. The origination of a 6.2 magnitude earthquake had been forecast; it happened at 09:03 on July 03, 1999. Due to the use of the claimed device its magnitude decreased by 0.8 points compared to the originally forecast magnitude.

Example 3. Under the conditions similar to example 1, a map of Alaska was scanned. The exact time of the origination of an earthquake with the magnitude of 4.8 had been forecast; it happened at 19:26 on July 4, 1999, and its magnitude decreased by 0.5 points.

Example 4. Under the conditions similar to example 1, a map of Philippines was scanned. The exact time of the earthquake with the magnitude of 4.0 had been forecast; it happened at 13:22 on July 4, 1999, and as the result of using the claimed device its magnitude decreased by 0.2 points.

Analysis of the obtained data demonstrates that complete confirmation of the forecasting phase was obtained 7 days before the beginning of an earthquake, with the exact indication of the time of the beginning of the earthquake. As a result of using the claimed device, the range of decrease magnitude was 0.2-0.8.

The advantages of the claimed method and the device for implementation thereof are increased efficiency due to accurate forecasting of the start of the origination of catastrophic phenomena, and the capability of remote normalization of the situation in zones of anticipated catastrophes. Used together, the claimed method and device have a broader field of application because they can be used for preparation for and prevention of both natural and anthropogenic catastrophes while completely maintaining environmental cleanliness when using them. Besides, the cost of implementation of the method is reduced due to the simplicity of its operations and the possibility of multiple use of the device by means of which the method is implemented.

CLAIMS

1.   A method for prevention of catastrophes comprising recording and processing of signals characterizing the situation in the zone of the anticipated catastrophe, distinct in that signals of light radiation from a component corresponding to the zone of the anticipated catastrophe are processed using an optical system comprised of sensory elements made of aligned crystals arranged in tandem along the direction of sensed

radiation, and normalized radiation for normalizing the situation in the zone of the anticipated catastrophe is formed in the optical system.

2. The method per claim 1, distinct in that continuous scanning of various sections of the component corresponding to the zone of the anticipated catastrophe is conducted, and the section of the origination of a catastrophe is identified by the increase of characteristics of radiation coming from the optical system compared to characteristics of radiation from other sections.

3. The method per claim 2, distinct in that the section of the origination of a natural catastrophe is identified by a 20-28% increase of characteristics of radiation corresponding to this section compared to characteristics of radiation from other sections.

4. The method per claim 2, distinct in that the section of the origination of an anthropogenic catastrophe is identified by a 10-12% increase of characteristics of radiation corresponding to this section compared to characteristics of radiation from other sections.

5. A device for prevention of catastrophes comprising a converter of signals characterizing the situation in the zone of the anticipated catastrophe, a signal recording system, and a radiator that generates signals facilitating normalization of the situation in this zone, distinct in that the signal converter comprises a component corresponding to the zone of the anticipated catastrophe, and an optical system comprising: sensory elements made from aligned crystals arranged in tandem along the direction of sensed light radiation and made in the form of identical cubes that are shifted with respect to each other and have different orientations of their optical axes, wherein respective planes of the cubes are parallel; a glass sphere wherein the cubes are located, the cubes and the sphere forming a continuous transparent structure; and a normalized radiation transducer connected to the last cube by means of an optical fiber, wherein the transducer is connected to a processor system that has a package of programs for processing the transducer signals.

6. The device per claim 5, distinct in that the signal transducer is made as a combination of the optical system and a map of the terrain where the origination of a catastrophic earthquake is anticipated.

7. The device per claim 5, distinct in that the signal transducer is made as a combination of the optical system and a telemetry system with a monitor where the component corresponding to the zone of an anticipated anthropogenic catastrophe is displayed.

8. The device per claim 5, distinct in that the processor system package of programs includes all kinds of parameters of zones of anticipated catastrophes.

NOTICES OF A CHANGE OF THE LEGAL STATUS

Code of change of the legal status   **MM4A**
Bulletin publication date   **2005.11.27**
Bulletin number   **200533**

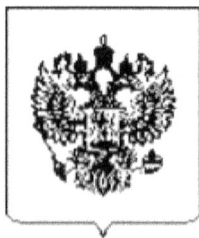

(19) **RU** (11) **2163419** (13) **C1**

(51) 7 H04B10/30

**FEDERAL SERVICE
FOR INTELLECTUAL PROPERTY,
PATENTS AND TRADEMARKS
(ROSPATENT)**

(12) DESCRIPTION OF THE PATENT
of the Russian Federation

(14) Publication date: 02.20.2001
(21) Application registration number: 2000117595/09
(22) Filing date: 07.06.2000
(24) Date of patent: 07.06.2000
(46) Date of publication of the claims: 02.20.2001
(56) Analogs of the invention: SU 2111617 A1,
05.20.1998. GRIGORI GRABOVOI "Исследование
и анализ фундаментальных определений
оптических систем для прогноза землетрясений
и катастроф производственного характера"
[The Study and Analysis of Fundamental Definitions
of Optical Systems for Forecasting Earthquakes and
Industrial Catastrophes], Moscow, RAEN Publishing
House, 1999, p. 9-19. BODYAKIN B.I. "Куда идешь,
человек? Основы эволюциологии" [Where Are
You Heading, Man? Fundamentals of Evolution
Studies], Moscow, SINTEG Publishing House, 1998,
p. 29-45, 79-95, 249.

(71) Applicant: **Grabovoi Grigori
Petrovich (aka Grigori Grabovoi®)**
(72) Inventor: **Grigori Grabovoi®**
(73) Patentee: **Grigori Grabovoi®**
(98) Address for correspondence: **115230,
Moscow, Kashirskoe Shosse
5-1-66, Kopaev, V.G.**

(54) AN INFORMATION TRANSMISISON SYSTEM

The invention relates to communication technology and can be used in wireless information transmission systems. The technical result is increased operational reliability and simultaneous increase of noise immunity. In the proposed system the signal transmitter comprises a sensing unit comprising spherical sensory elements made of glass and rigidly secured by means of glue joints to a supporting member, and a spherical module installed on it made in the form of a glass sphere inside which the sensory elements in the form of identical cubes made of crystal are secured. The signal receiver is distanced from the transmitter and comprises a sensing unit and a spherical module distanced from it that are similar to the respective components, and the spherical module has a device for converting radiation to output signals. Diameters of all sensory elements that are part of the sensing unit should differ from each other, for instance, they should

42

increase gradually. When transmitting information, the operator activates the sensory elements of the signal transmitter. Then, practically instantly, the activation radiation is reproduced in the sensory elements of the signal transmitter and normalized by the sensory elements of the spherical module. The transducer converts output normalized radiation to electric signals, and after processing in the processor the transmitted information arrives at a recorder.

DESCRIPTION OF THE INVENTION

The invention relates to the field of communication technology and can be used in information transmission systems that use wireless communication between the transmitter and receiver, mainly when transmitting information over considerable (thousands of kilometers) distances.

The closest to the claimed system in the technical essence is the information transmission system comprising a transmission unit with a supporting member with signal transmitters rigidly attached to, and a distanced from it receiving unit comprising a supporting member with signal receivers rigidly secured to it, and a device that converts radiation to output signals (see RF Patent No. 2111617, cl. H 04 B 10/00). In the known system, laser beams are used as communication channels between the transmitter and the receiver. Each signal transmitter is made in the form of a laser generator with a device for modulating the laser beam by a data signal connected to the source of data signals. Each signal receiver is made in the form of a photo detector and a device converting sensed laser-modulated radiation to electrical data signals.

The shortcoming of the known system is low operational reliability due to design complexity of the system with its large number of complex data transmitters and receivers with multifunctional links and complex precision pointing systems with movable components. In the known system, when transmitting information between the signal transmitter and receiver located at a considerable distance from each other, for instance, when transmitting information over thousands of kilometers using a spacecraft with a repeater, information transmission delay can equal several tenths of one second. The known system does not have sufficient noise immunity because when there is an obstacle in the laser communication line there is interference in the system operation or a breakdown of transmitted signals.

The invention object is to increase operational reliability of the information transmission system while ensuring transmission of information without delay and increasing the system noise immunity. Said object is achieved by the new information transmission system comprising a signal transmitter and signal receiver a distanced from it, each comprising a sensing unit in the form of spherical sensory elements having different diameters and rigidly secured on the surface of a supporting member, and a spherical module in the form of a glass sphere with sensory elements in the form of identical cubes secured inside it. The sensory elements are made of crystal and distributed along the same direction, and shifted with respect to each other in two mutually perpendicular planes; the transmitter elements are similar to the receiver elements, the spherical module of the signal transmitter is located on the surface of the supporting member, and the spherical module of the signal receiver is distanced from its sensing unit and has a device for converting radiation to output signals.

Herein, it is preferable to: uniformly distribute the spherical sensory elements over the surface of the supporting member and to place centers of the elements in parallel planes; make on the surface of the supporting member of the signal transmitter near each spherical sensory element an image of a certain letter of all letters of the alphabet, or an image of a certain number of the entire series of natural numbers, or an image of a symbol; place the spherical sensory elements on the surface of the supporting member in identical rows; make the spherical sensory elements with gradually increasing diameters; make the device for converting radiation to output signals in the form of a transducer connected by means of an optical fiber to the spherical module cube located the farthest from the sensing unit of the radiation receiver; connect the

The invention is based on the similarity principle that has been established by the author and is based on the theory of wave synthesis developed by the author, combined with the formula of general formula (see the thesis for the degree of a Doctor of Physical and Mathematical Sciences: Grigori Grabovoi, "Исследование и анализ фундаментальных определений оптических систем для прогноза землетрясений и катастроф производственных объектов" [Research and Analysis of Basic Definitions of Optical Systems for Forecasting Earthquakes and Catastrophes of Industrial Facilities], Moscow, RAEN Publishing House, 1999, pp. 9 - 19).

According to the theory of wave synthesis, reality can be viewed as a periodic intersection of stationary and dynamic regions, wherein the synthesis of a dynamic wave and a stationary wave occurs in the intersection zones. Any phenomenon of reality can be defined in the form of optical systems, and because a person's perception is realized by means of images – light elements that contain information, information transmission at the first stage from the person generating the transmitted information to a person's information-sensing optical sensory element can be viewed as a peculiar optical transmission system. Transmitted information generated by human operator's thoughts is received by an optical sensory element the operator aims the generated thought at.

Known are various optical devices, for instance, a "Камера-3000" camera that makes it possible to record a change of person's aura (see Komkov, V.N., "Сенсоры биополя и ауры" [The Biologic Field and Aura Sensors], "Электронная техника, серия 3, Микроэлектроника", 1999, vol. 1(153), p. 23). Because thought is part of aura, it too can be transmitted in the form of an element of a "weak" optical system. It is preferable to make the information-sensing sensory element in the shape of a sphere because it is precisely the spherical shape of the sensory element that facilitates maximum activation of the sensory element due to internal reflection. The radiation of activated spherical sensory elements is light radiation, and each operator who transmits information will have the corresponding individual characteristics of the radiation which determines the high noise immunity of the claimed system. Individual activation of spherical sensory elements is achieved due to the use of a set of such elements that have different diameters, which determines the difference of radiation emitted by different elements. It is preferable to use a set of spherical sensory elements with gradually increasing diameters. The number of spherical sensory elements in a set can vary. It is preferable to choose the number of elements in a set equal to the sum of letters in the alphabet and the sum of figures in the series of natural numbers.

All spherical sensory elements in a set of such elements are rigidly secured to the surface of the supporting member made, for instance, in the shape of a plate. The supporting member and spherical sensory elements secured on its surface form a sensing unit. The signal transmitter and signal receiver have

44

similar sensing units, which ensures reproduction of the transferred information.

It follows from the theory of wave synthesis and quantum mechanics laws that thought converted to radiation can have two quantum states at the same time (see Grigori Grabovoi, "Исследования и анализ фундаментальных определений оптических систем в предотвращении катастроф и прогнозно-ориентированном управлении микропроцессорами" [The Study and Analysis of Fundamental Definitions of Optical Systems in Preventing Catastrophes and Forecast-Oriented Microprocessors' Management], "Электронная техника, серия 3, Микроэлектроника", 1999, vol. 1 (153), p. 10). One of these states is on a sensory element of the signal transmitter, and the other one is on a similar sensory element of the signal receiver. To facilitate the work of a human operator who generates transmitted information, it is preferable to uniformly distribute spherical sensing elements over the surface of the supporting member and to locate the centers of spherical sensory elements in parallel planes, as well as to arrange these centers in identical rows.

Besides, on the surface of the supporting member of the signal transmitter near each spherical sensory element an image of a corresponding letter of the alphabet, of a figure or of a certain symbol is made. Along with using at the first stage transmission of information by means of spherical sensory elements one can also use a spherical module with arranged in tandem sensory elements in the form of identical cubes made of crystal secured inside. At a certain mutual arrangement of the cubes, normalization of radiation initiated by human operator's thought and characterizing a combination of certain letters of a word will occur.

In accordance with the similarity principle, at the second stage of information transmission radiation emitted by a spherical sensory element is reproduced practically instantly, with no delay, in a similar spherical sensory element in the sensing unit of the signal receiver. Then radiation arrives at the spherical module of the signal receiver made similarly to the spherical module of the signal transmitter. The spherical module of the signal receiver is made in the form of a glass sphere, with sensory elements in the form of identical cubes made of crystal, distributed along the same direction and shifted with respect to each other in two mutually perpendicular planes secured inside.

After being received at the first cube which is the closest to the receiver sensing unit, initial normalization of radiation by the first cube will occur at the moment when radiation exiting from the third cube passes through the fourth cube. The next normalization act occurs when radiation passes through all cubes. Light has been selected as the information-carrying medium because this makes it possible to visualize and record the laws of relations established by the formula of general reality. After normalization in the spherical module of the signal receiver, radiation emitted by a spherical sensory element of the signal receiver exits the cube that is the farthest from the receiver sensing unit; herein, the amount of exiting normalized radiation depends on the diameter of the spherical sensory element of the signal transmitter the spherical sensory element of the signal receiver is similar to.

The sensing unit and the spherical module of the signal transmitter are made similar to the respective components of the signal receiver; however, they can have different geometric dimensions. Thus, geometric dimensions of elements of the signal receiver can be 3-5 times as large as the corresponding dimensions of the signal transmitter. As a device that converts radiation exiting the last cube one can use an optical converter in the form of a radiation receiver and a microprocessor that converts radiation intensity to digital data, or a normalized radiation transducer connected to the last cube by means of an optical fiber and connected via an electric signal amplifier to a programmable control processor.

The attached drawings show the following: Fig. 1 shows the general view of the information transmission system (isometric view), Fig. 2 shows the sensing unit (front view), and Fig. 3 shows an individual spherical element rigidly secured on the supporting member.

The claimed information transmission system comprises a sensing unit 1 of the signal receiver [sic] comprising a supporting member 2, with spherical sensory elements 3 rigidly secured on it and uniformly distributed over its surface; a spherical module 4 of the signal transmitter comprising a glass sphere 5 with sensory elements 6 in the form of identical cubes secured in it; a sensing unit 7 of the signal receiver which is similar to the analogous unit of the signal transmitter and also comprises a supporting member 8 and spherical sensory elements 9 rigidly secured on it; a spherical module 10 of the signal receiver which is similar to the analogous unit of the signal transmitter and also comprises a glass sphere 11 with sensory elements 12 in the form of identical cubes secured in it; a normalized radiation transducer 13, with an amplifier 14 connected to it, the amplifier is connected to the input of programmed control processor 15, and display 16 and recorder 17 are connected to the processor; herein, each spherical sensory element is rigidly secured to the supporting member surface by means of fastener 18.

It is preferable to make the spherical sensory elements 3 and 9 from a transparent material, for instance, from glass. Diameters of all sensory elements of a sensing unit, for instance, of the signal receiver unit 1, must be different from each other, each diameter corresponding to a certain letter, figure or symbol. It is preferable that the diameter increase gradually, for instance, from 1 to 53 mm. Similarly, diameters of all spherical sensory elements 9 of the sensing unit 7 of the signal receiver must also be different from each other. Each spherical sensory element is rigidly secured to the surface of the respective supporting member by means of fastener 18, for instance, by means of a glue joint. It is preferable to place spherical sensory elements in identical rows on the supporting member surface (see Fig. 2; some elements not shown) wherein element diameters increase gradually in each row.

Fig. 1

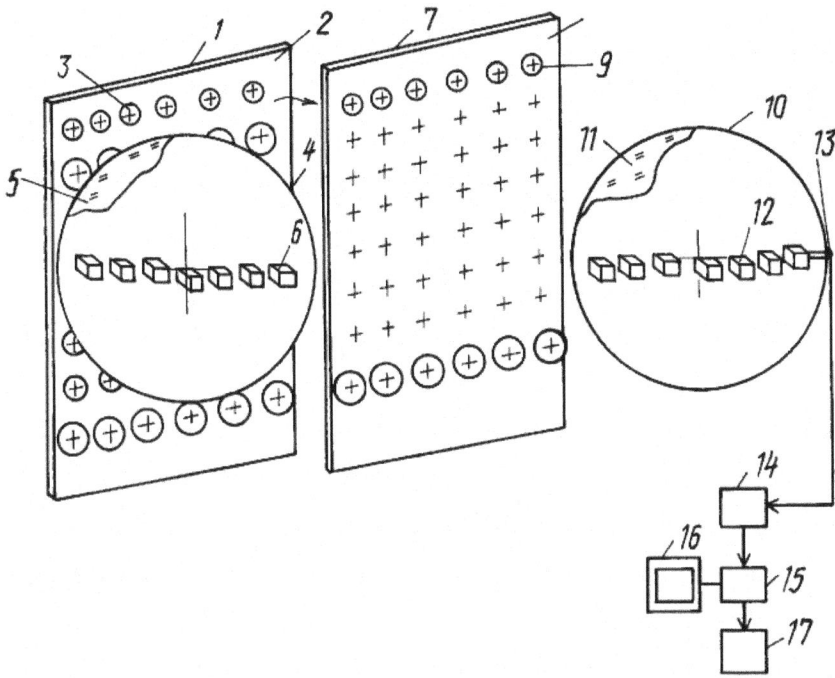

Fig. 2

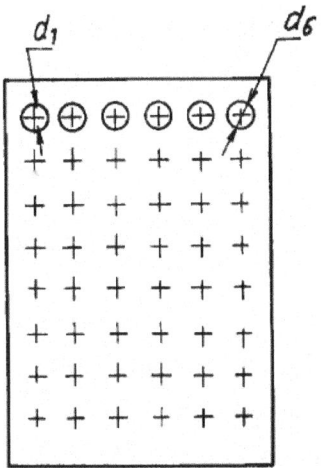

Fig3

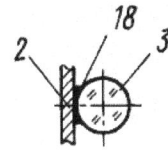

47

Each spherical module 4 or 10 (see Fig. 1) comprises a glass sphere. For instance, the spherical module 4 of the signal transmitter comprises the glass sphere 5, inside which sensory elements 6 in the form of identical cubes distributed along a straight line perpendicular to the surface of the supporting member 2 are secured and form a monolithic system with the sphere. The number of cubes can be 7, 14, etc. Usually, seven cubes are used. Cubes 6 or 12 are made from crystal, for instance, from diamond or rock crystal. The cubes are located in the spherical module in tandem, with different orientation of their optical axes. The faces of adjacent cubes are parallel, and the cubes themselves are shifted with respect to each other in two mutually perpendicular planes. It is preferable to place the spherical module 4 of the signal transmitter in the center of the supporting member 2. The spherical module 10 of the signal receiver is distanced from the sensing unit 7, preferably by 200-1000 mm.

The claimed information transmission system works as follows. The operator (not shown) transmitting information is a person who generates a thought. In 0.1-5 s (the time depends on the person's bioenergy field) the operator activates sensory elements 3 of the sensing unit 1 of the signal transmitter. Signals coming from the operator's optical system are amplified by spherical sensory elements 3 of the signal transmitter and with no delay, practically instantly, reproduced in respective sensory elements 9 of the signal receiver, wherein a signal transmitted by an element 3 of the transmitter is reproduced by a similar element 9 of the receiver, in accordance with the similarity principle. Then radiation of sensory elements 9 of the signal receiver is converted by sensory elements 12 of the spherical module 10 of the signal receiver. The amount of transmitted information corresponds to the amount of information contained in the generated optical image. For instance, after information contained in a CD reader is perceived by the operator it can be transmitted completely to the signal receiver.

When radiation passes through elements 12 in the form of cubes, normalization of the form of light volume determined by mutual location of the cubes takes place. Here, for each diameter of a spherical sensory element 9 there is a corresponding amount of normalized radiation coming from the cube 12 that is farthest away from the sensing unit 8 of the signal receiver. Normalized radiation coming out from this cube is transmitted through the optical fiber to the normalized radiation transducer 13, and after passing through the amplifier 14 electric signals coming from the transducer arrive at the programmable control processor 15. Signals processed in the processor 15 that correspond to the transmitted information in the form of letters, figures and/or symbols can be displayed on the display 16 and arrive at the recording device 17 which can have modules for recording and storage of incoming information for subsequent processing.

Compared to the known system the claimed system has much higher operational reliability because the claimed system design has been maximally simplified and there are no moving elements. Unlike the known system, the claimed system provides information transmission over considerable (thousands of kilometers) distances with no delays. Besides, the claimed system has higher noise immunity because obstacles located between its receiver and transmitter do not interfere with transmission of information.

CLAIMS

1.   An information transmission system comprising a signal transmitter and a signal receiver distanced from it, each comprising a sensing unit in the form of spherical optical sensory elements that have different diameters and are rigidly secured on the surface of a supporting member, and a spherical module in the form of a glass sphere inside which optical sensory elements in the form of identical cubes made of rock crystal or diamond are secured, the sensory elements are spread along the same direction and shifted with respect to each other in two mutually perpendicular planes, wherein the transmitter elements are similar to the receiver elements, the module of the transmitter is located on the surface of the supporting member of its sensing unit, optical sensory elements of the transmitter sense transmitted information generated by the operator, and the spherical module of the signal receiver is distanced from its sensing unit and connected to the device for converting radiation to output signals.

2.   The system per claim 1, distinct in that the spherical optical sensory elements are uniformly distributed over the surface of the supporting member, and the centers of these elements are located in parallel planes.

3.   The system per claim 1 or 2, distinct in that an image of a certain letter of all letters of the alphabet, or of a certain figure of the entire series of natural numbers, or of a certain symbol with an arbitrary shape is made on the surface of the supporting member of the signal transmitter near each spherical optical sensory element.

4.   The system per claim 1, distinct in that the spherical optical sensory elements are located on the surface of the supporting member in identical rows.

5.   The system per any of the above claims, distinct in that the diameters of various optical sensory elements increase gradually.

6.   The system per claim 1, distinct in that the supporting member surface is located orthogonally to the direction of distribution of the spherical module cubes.

NOTICES OF A CHANGE OF THE LEGAL STATUS

Code of change of the legal status	**MM4A**
Bulletin publication date	**2005.04.20**
Bulletin number	**200511**

СЕРТИФИКАТ-ЛИЦЕНЗИЯ

Регистрационный номер№ 000283   Шифр 00012   Код 00015

Открытие, изобретение, новшество (технология, проект и т.д.): **МЕТОД**

Грабовой Григорий Петрович

Аннотация:

Разработана технология перевода информации любого события в геометрические формы описываемые ортодоксальной математикой. Для изменения события специальная компьютерная программа, первоначальную форму переводит в форму изменяющую событие необходимым образом. Программа основана на расчетах угловых коэффициентов между измененными и дополненными формами, т.е. рассчитывается четырехкратный интеграл методом Рунге-Кутта. Дополненные формы при специальном импульсе управляют на любом расстоянии. Использование компьютерной технологии может быть полезно в управлении информацией в медицине, в точных технологиях и др.

Краткое название: КОМПЬЮТЕРНАЯ ТЕХНОЛОГИЯ ДИСТАНТНОГО УПРАВЛЕНИЯ

Основная идея:

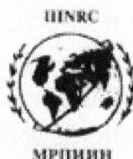

Международная регистрационная палата информационно-интеллектуальной новизны представляет на регистрацию в Международный Регистр Глобальных Систем Информации интеллектуальную собственность, которая, как творческая работа, была признана Ученым Советом МРПИИН и другими структурами как

МЕТОД

Настоящий Сертификат-Лицензия - документ, дающий владельцу право использовать эту информационно-интеллектуальную новизну, как собственность, на международных рынках всех стран Мира.

Председатель Палаты,
действительный член Международной
Академии информатизации и
Нью-Йоркской Академии наук

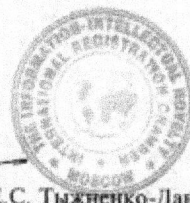

Е.С. Тыжненко-Давтян

Дата: 19 декабря 1997

INTERNATIONAL INFORMATIONAL INTELLECTUAL NOVELTY
REGISTRATION CHAMBER
EMBLEM
CERTIFICATE-LICENSE

Registration No 000283   Cipher 00012   Code 00015

Discovery, invention, novelty (technology, project, etc.)   **METHOD**

GRABOVOI GRIGORI PETROVICH

Abstract:

A process has been developed for converting information of any event to geometric forms described by orthodox mathematics. To change an event, a special computer program converts the original form to a form that changes the event the required way. The program is based on computation of angular coefficients between the changed and amended forms, i.e. the Runge-Kutta quadruple integral is computed. With a special pulse, amended forms control at any distance. The use of computer technology can be helpful in controlling information in medicine, in precision technologies, etc.

Short title: A COMPUTER TECHNOLOGY OF REMOTE CONTROL

Main idea:

The International Information Intellectual Novelty Registration Chamber hereby presents to the International Register of Global Information Systems, for registration, the intellectual property which, as a creative work, has been recognized by the IIINRC Scientific Council and by other structures as a

METHOD

This Certificate-License is a document granting the holder the right to use this informational-intellectual novelty as a property in the international markets of all the World countries.

S/Chamber Chairman, Member of the International Academy of Informatization
  (in good standing) and New York Academy of Sciences
  Ye.S.Tyzhnenko-Davtyan   [Signature]

L.S. [Official Round Seal]

Date: December 19, 1997

СЕРТИФИКАТ-ЛИЦЕНЗИЯ

Регистрационный номер№ 000285   Шифр 00014   Код 00015

Открытие, изобретение, новшество (технология, проект и т.д.): **МОДЕЛЬ**

Грабовой Григорий Петрович

Аннотация:

Новизна в принципах расщепления информации, основанной на постулатах общности пространства и времени в бесконечности и принципах сочетания известных свойств пространства и времени с законами их взаимного развития. Открыт метод архивации любой информации через область бесконечно удаленных точек. Пространство рассматривается как неизменяемая структура времени. Время рассматривается как функция пространства, а точка воспроизводства материи как следствие реакции времени на изменение пространства. Точки соприкосновения и являются точками архивации любой информации, что позволяет создать технологические системы на основе ЭВМ. Заархивированная информация дает статичную конструкцию машины «разумной» и процессы управления ею. Можно также заархивировать информацию в любом веществе непрерывной записью и считать ее информацией не имеющей видимого материального носителя. Таким вариантом применяемой модели архивации можно создать принципиально новый вид компьютерной техники, которая может быть использована для создания необходимой формы разума, находящегося в воздухе, в вакууме или в любом веществе, через единичные импульсы специальной приставки к компьютеру.

Краткое название: АРХИВАЦИЯ ИНФОРМАЦИИ В ЛЮБОЙ ТОЧКЕ ПРОСТРАНСТВА-ВРЕМЕНИ

Основная идея:

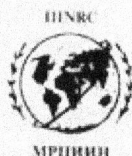

Международная регистрационная палата информационно-интеллектуальной новизны представляет на регистрацию в Международный Регистр Глобальных Систем Информации интеллектуальную собственность, которая, как творческая работа, была признана Ученым Советом МРПИИН и другими структурами как

МОДЕЛЬ

Настоящий Сертификат-Лицензия - документ, дающий владельцу право использовать эту информационно-интеллектуальную новизну, как собственность, на международных рынках всех стран Мира.

Председатель Палаты,
действительный член Международной
Академии информатизации и
Нью-Йоркской Академии наук

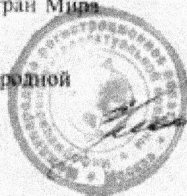

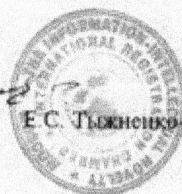

Е.С. Тыжненко-Давтян

Дата: 19 декабря 1997

INTERNATIONAL INFORMATIONAL INTELLECTUAL NOVELTY REGISTRATION CHAMBER
EMBLEM
CERTIFICATE-LICENSE

Registration No 000285   Cipher 00014   Code 00015

Discovery, invention, novelty (technology, project, etc.)   **MODEL**

GRABOVOI GRIGORI PETROVICH

Abstract:

Novelty is in principles of splitting information that is based on postulates of the commonality of space and time in infinity and on principles of combining the known properties of space and time with the laws of their mutual development. A method has been discovered for archiving any information via a field of infinitely remote points. The space is regarded as a fixed structure of time. Time is regarded as a function of space, and the point of reproduction of matter is regarded as the consequence of time response to a change of space. Points of contiguity are the points of archiving any information, which makes it possible to create computer-based technology systems. Archived information makes "intelligent" the static structure of a machine and the methods to control the machine. It is also possible to archive information in any substance by means of continuous recording and to regard it as information that has no visible material medium. With this version of the applied archiving model it is possible to create a fundamentally new type of computer technology that can be used to create the required form of intelligence located in air, in vacuum or in any substance by using unit pulses of a special attachment to a computer.

Short title: ARCHIVING INFORMATION AT ANY SPACE-TIME POINT

Main idea:

The International Information Intellectual Novelty Registration Chamber hereby presents to the International Register of Global Information Systems, for registration, the intellectual property which, as a creative work, has been recognized by the IIINRC Scientific Council and by other structures as a

MODEL

This Certificate-License is a document granting the holder the right to use this informational-intellectual novelty as a property in the international markets of all the World countries.

S/Chamber Chairman, Member of the International Academy of Informatization (in good standing) and New York Academy of Sciences
Ye.S.Tyzhnenko-Davtyan   [Signature]

L.S. [Official Round Seal]

Date: December 19, 1997

INTERNATIONAL
INFORMATION
INTELLECTUAL NOVELTY
REGISTRATION CHAMBER

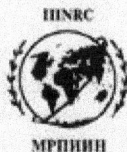

IIINRC

МРПИИН

МЕЖДУНАРОДНАЯ
РЕГИСТРАЦИОННАЯ ПАЛАТА
ИНФОРМАЦИОННО-
ИНТЕЛЛЕКТУАЛЬНОЙ
НОВИЗНЫ

СЕРТИФИКАТ-ЛИЦЕНЗИЯ

Регистрационный номер№ 000287   Шифр 00018   Код 00015

Открытие, изобретение, новшество (технология, проект и т.д.): **ОТКРЫТИЕ**

Грабовой Григорий Петрович

Аннотация:

Предложены новые области информации, определяющие свойства и места расположения любых объектов информации приводящих к саморазвитию неразрушающих областей созидания, определяющих также конкретные технологии неразрушающего использования создающей области. Открыта полная идентичность (по принципу аутоморфности, изоморфичности) любых объектов информации перед создающей областью информации (протоколы результатов заверены нотариально в ООН).

Открытие создающей области информации осуществилось через отражение реализуемых объектов информации на внутренней поверхности сферы прошлых (известных) объектов информации. Сегмент сферы соответствующей будущей информации определяющий компоненты создаваемых объектов , находится как площадь внешней поверхности сферы известных объектов информации, определяемая из проекций областей реализуемых объектов на внешнюю поверхность сферы известных объектов и возникает из взаимодействия областей информации критериально идентичных, по отношению к создающей области, через внутренние области динамичных, по отношению к объектам реализации, сфер. Открытие позволяет реализовать любые направления созидательного развития по принципу самопостижения с применением метода ортодоксальной математики.

Краткое название: ВОСПРОИЗВОДЯЩИЕ САМОРАЗВИВАЮЩИЕСЯ СИСТЕМЫ, ОТРАЖАЮЩИЕ ВНЕШНИЕ И ВНУТРЕНИЕ ОБЛАСТИ МНОГООБРАЗИЯ СОЗДАЮЩИХ СФЕР

Основная идея:

Международная регистрационная палата информационно-интеллектуальной новизны представляет на регистрацию в Международный Регистр Глобальных Систем Информации интеллектуальную собственность, которая, как творческая работа, была признана Ученым Советом МРПИИН и другими структурами как

ОТКРЫТИЕ

Настоящий Сертификат-Лицензия - документ, дающий владельцу право использовать эту информационно-интеллектуальную новизну, как собственность, на международных рынках всех стран Мира.

Председатель Палаты,
действительный член Международной
Академии информатизации и
Нью-Йоркской Академии наук

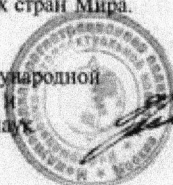

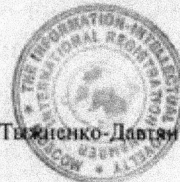

Е.С. Тихоненко-Давтян

Дата: 19 декабря 1997

INTERNATIONAL INFORMATIONAL INTELLECTUAL NOVELTY REGISTRATION CHAMBER
EMBLEM
CERTIFICATE-LICENSE

Registration No 000287   Cipher 00018   Code 00015

Discovery, invention, novelty (technology, project, etc.)   **DISCOVERY**

GRABOVOI GRIGORI PETROVICH

Abstract:

New fields of information have been proposed that determine the properties and location of any object of information leading to self-development of non-destructive fields of creation and that also determine specific technologies of non-destructive use of the creating field. Complete equivalence (based on the principle of automorphism and isomorphism) of any objects of information before the creating field of information has been discovered (the results reports were notarized at the UN).

The discovery of the creating field of information was accomplished through reflection of realizable objects of information on the inner surface of the sphere of past (known) objects of information. The sphere segment of the relevant future information that defines components of the created objects is determined as the area of the outer surface of the sphere of known objects of information which is determined from projections of fields of realizable objects on the outer surface of the sphere of known objects and originates from the interaction of information fields that are identical, criterion-wise, with respect to the creating field, via inner fields of spheres that are dynamic with respect to objects of realization. The discovery makes it possible to realize any directions of creative development according to the principle of self-comprehension using the orthodox mathematics method.

Short title: REPRODUCTIVE SELFDEVELOPING SYSTEMS REFLECTING THE OUTER AND INNER FIELDS OF THE VARIETY OF CREATING SPHERES

Main idea:

The International Information Intellectual Novelty Registration Chamber hereby presents to the International Register of Global Information Systems, for registration, the intellectual property which, as a creative work, has been recognized by the IIINRC Scientific Council and by other structures as a

DISCOVERY

This Certificate-License is a document granting the holder the right to use this informational-intellectual novelty as a property in the international markets of all the World countries.

**S/Chamber Chairman, Member of the International Academy of Informatization (in good standing) and New York Academy of Sciences
Ye.S.Tyzhnenko-Davtyan   [Signature]**

L.S. [Official Round Seal]

Date: December 19, 1997

INTERNATIONAL
INFORMATION
INTELLECTUAL NOVELTY
REGISTRATION CHAMBER

IINRC

МРПИИН

МЕЖДУНАРОДНАЯ
РЕГИСТРАЦИОННАЯ ПАЛАТА
ИНФОРМАЦИОННО-
ИНТЕЛЛЕКТУАЛЬНОЙ
НОВИЗНЫ

СЕРТИФИКАТ-ЛИЦЕНЗИЯ

Регистрационный номер№ 000286   Шифр 00020   Код 00015

Открытие, изобретение, новшество (технология, проект и т.д.): **ПРИНЦИП**

Грабовой Григорий Петрович

Аннотация:

Открыто свойство материи позволяющая практически мгновенно получать необходимую форму на основе единичной программы заложенной в какой либо интервал времени (имеются протокольные доказательства). Компьютерные технологии позволяют обеспечить управление материей, восстановление тканей организма и его безопасность, контроль за машинами, создание вещества принципом перевода времени в любое вещество - принципом не разрушаемости структуры времени при изменении пространства; источник энергии из времени прошлых событий неограничен, т.е. любое событие прошлого можно дробить бесконечным количеством методов, в т.ч. и методом обратной связи - управление временем будущих событий. Фактически при применении прикладного аппарата на концептуальной основе, можно использовать время прошлых событий. Следовательно, по мнению автора восстановить можно любую материю из набора «случайных» событий в любом интервале времени, что означает нелогичность любого разрушения.

Краткое название: ВРЕМЯ, ЭТО ФОРМА ПРОСТРАНСТВА

Основная идея:

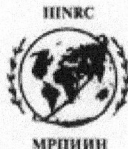

Международная регистрационная палата информационно-интеллектуальной новизны представляет на регистрацию в Международный Регистр Глобальных Систем Информации интеллектуальную собственность, которая, как творческая работа, была признана Ученым Советом МРПИИН и другими структурами как

ПРИНЦИП

Настоящий Сертификат-Лицензия - документ, дающий владельцу право использовать эту информационно-интеллектуальную новизну, как собственность, на международных рынках всех стран Мира.

Председатель Палаты,
действительный член Международной
Академии информатизации и
Нью-Йоркской Академии наук

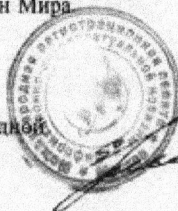

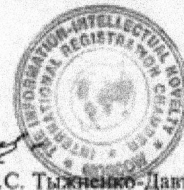

Е.С. Тыжненко-Давтян

Дата: 19 декабря 1997

INTERNATIONAL INFORMATIONAL INTELLECTUAL NOVELTY REGISTRATION CHAMBER
EMBLEM
CERTIFICATE-LICENSE

Registration No 000286   Cipher 00020   Code 00015
Discovery, invention, novelty (technology, project, etc.)   **PRINCIPLE**

GRABOVOI GRIGORI PETROVICH

Abstract:

A property of matter has been discovered that makes it possible to practically instantly derive the required form based on the unit program embedded into a time interval (records of proof are available). Computer technologies make it possible to ensure control of matter, repair of body tissues, body safety, control of machines, creation of substance using the principle of converting time to any substance – the principle of indestructibility of the structure of time when space changes; the source of energy from the time of past events is unlimited, i.e. any event of the past can be split using infinite number of methods, including the feedback method – controlling the time of future events. Actually, when using the application apparatus on a conceptual base it is possible to use the time of past events. Therefore, in the author's opinion it is possible to restore any matter from a set of "random" events, which means the illogicality of any destruction.

Short title: TIME IS A FORM OF SPACE

Main idea:

The International Information Intellectual Novelty Registration Chamber hereby presents to the International Register of Global Information Systems, for registration, the intellectual property which, as a creative work, has been recognized by the IIINRC Scientific Council and by other structures as a

PRINCIPLE

This Certificate-License is a document granting the holder the right to use this informational-intellectual novelty as a property in the international markets of all the World countries.

S/Chamber Chairman, Member of the International Academy of Informatization (in good standing) and New York Academy of Sciences
Ye.S.Tyzhnenko-Davtyan   [Signature]

L.S. [Official Round Seal]
Date: December 19, 1997

СЕРТИФИКАТ-ЛИЦЕНЗИЯ

Регистрационный номер№ 000284   Шифр 00020   Код 00015

Открытие, изобретение, новшество (технология, проект и т.д.): **ПРИНЦИП**

Грабовой Григорий Петрович

Аннотация:

Перевод атласа морфологии человека в геометрическую форму дает возможность диагностировать объект в реальном времени на основании видео, фотографии, почерка, инициалов и т.п. При этом можно знать всю гистологию не проводя срезов тканей, пункций и т.п. Метод позволяет на принципиальной основе определять опасные состояния организма, контролировать на расстоянии жизнедеятельность и возможности ее восстановления в определенных случаях. Переводится также любой иной объект в геометрическую форму посредством цифровой обработки знаний о состоянии, трубо-нефтепроводов, скважин, катастрофах природного и технического характера. Диагностируются также неисправности и отклонения от технических условий эксплуатации машин в прошлом, настоящем и будущем времени.

Краткое название: ДИАГНОСТИКА ОБЪЕКТА МЕТОДАМИ ОРТОДОКСАЛЬНОЙ МАТЕМАТИКИ

Основная идея:

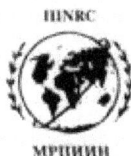

Международная регистрационная палата информационно-интеллектуальной новизны представляет на регистрацию в Международный Регистр Глобальных Систем Информации интеллектуальную собственность, которая, как творческая работа, была признана Ученым Советом МРПИИН и другими структурами как

ПРИНЦИП

Настоящий Сертификат-Лицензия - документ, дающий владельцу право использовать эту информационно-интеллектуальную новизну, как собственность, на международных рынках всех стран Мира.

Председатель Палаты,
действительный член Международной
Академии информатизации и
Нью-Йоркской Академии наук   Е.С. Тыжненко-Давтян

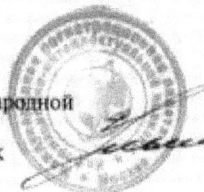

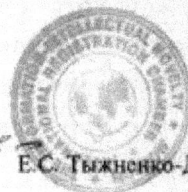

Дата: 19 декабря 1997

INTERNATIONAL INFORMATIONAL INTELLECTUAL NOVELTY REGISTRATION CHAMBER
EMBLEM
CERTIFICATE-LICENSE

Registration No 000284   Cipher 00020   Code 00015

Discovery, invention, novelty (technology, project, etc.)   **PRINCIPLE**

GRABOVOI GRIGORI PETROVICH

Abstract:

Conversion of person's morphology atlas to geometric form makes it possible to diagnose the object in real time based on a video, a photograph, handwriting, initials, etc. Furthermore, it is possible to know all histology without performing tissue section, punctures, etc. The method makes it possible on the principle basis to determine body's dangerous states, to remotely control vital activity and the possibilities of restoring it in certain cases. Also, any object is converted to geometric form by means of digital processing of knowledge of the state of oil pipelines, wells, and of knowledge of natural and anthropogenic catastrophes. Also diagnosed are malfunctions and deviations from operational specifications of machines in past, present and future time.

Short title: DIAGNOSTICS OF AN OBJECT USING THE METHODS OF ORTHODOX MATHEMATICS

Main idea:

The International Information Intellectual Novelty Registration Chamber hereby presents to the International Register of Global Information Systems, for registration, the intellectual property which, as a creative work, has been recognized by the IIINRC Scientific Council and by other structures as a

PRINCIPLE

This Certificate-License is a document granting the holder the right to use this informational-intellectual novelty as a property in the international markets of all the World countries.

S/Chamber Chairman, Member of the International Academy of Informatization
   (in good standing) and New York Academy of Sciences
   Ye.S.Tyzhnenko-Davtyan   [Signature]

L.S. [Official Round Seal]

Date: December 19, 1997

INTERNATIONAL INFORMATIZATION ACADEMY

in the Consultative Status (Category I) with the Economic and Social Council of United Nations

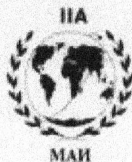

IIA
МАИ

IINIRC
МРПИИН

INTERNATIONAL INFORMATION INTELLECTUAL NOVELTY REGISTRATION CHAMBER

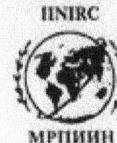

CERTIFICATE-LICENCE

Registration № EIW 000287   Cipher 00018   Code 0015

Discovery, invention, innovation (technology, project, etc.): **DISCIVERIES**

Grigory P. Grabovoi

Information summary:

New information areas are discovered, which define properties and locations of any information items leading to self-development of non-destructible areas of creative activity, and define particular technologies of non-destructive use of a creative area. It was discovered that any information items are completely identical (with the underlying principles of automorphism and isomorphism) to the creative information area (the outcome protocols are certified by the notary in the U. N.).

Commonality-creating information was discovered through reflections of real information items on the interior surface of the sphere of past (known) information items. A segment of the sphere of respective future information, which determines the components of items being created, is defined as the square of outer surface of the sphere of known information items; this square is derived from projections made from areas of real items to the outer surface of the sphere of known items; it comes from interaction of information areas (which are criteria-identical to the creating area) through internal areas which are dynamic in relation to information items. The above discovery makes it possible to activate any creative development areas, on the basis of the self-comprehension principle, by using orthodox mathematics methods.

A method is developed to diagnose objects. Programs are based on computer-aided distant management technologies which allow archiving information in any point of space-time.

A brief title: REPRODUCING SELF-EVOLVING SYSTEMS REFLECTING EXTERNAL AND INTERNAL AREAS OF A VARIETY OF CREATING SPHERES

International Informatization Academy (IIA) and International Registration Chamber submit to the International register of the Global Automatization Information Systems intellectual property, (either personal or party) which, as creative work, has been recognized by government and other structures as a

DISCOVERIES

for its realization in investments markets worldwide under obligations described in the contract- agreement made with the owner(s) of the Certificate - Licence.

The Certificate - Licence is the document which permits its owner(s) to get payment for the right to use this intellectual property in the international markets.

E. Tyzhnenko-Davtian
Chairman Registration
Chamber, Vice-President of IIA,
Academician

Date: December 24, 1997

Series MO
Register #00287

Headquarters: New York, Washington, Geneva, Montreal, Moscow

GRIGORI GRABOVOI

PATENTS FOR INVENTIONS

ISBN: 978-3-00-034093-2

GRIGORI GRABOVOI

PATENTS FOR INVENTIONS

EDITION: 2011-2, 05.07.2011

Hamburg 2011